THE QUEST FOR WELLNESS

A PRACTICAL & PERSONAL WELLNESS PLAN FOR
OPTIMUM HEALTH IN YOUR BODY, MIND EMOTIONS & SPIRIT

MARK SHERWOOD, ND
WITH
MICHELE NEIL-SHERWOOD, DO

emerge
publishing

TULSA, OKLAHOMA

17 16 15 14   10 9 8 7 6 5 4 3 2 1

THE QUEST FOR WELLNESS — A Practical and Personal Wellness Plan for Optimum Health in your Body, Mind, Emotions and Spirit.

TULSA, OKLAHOMA

Published by:
Emerge Publishing, LLC
9521B Riverside Parkway, Suite 243
Tulsa, Oklahoma 74137
Phone: 888.407.4447
www.EmergePublishing.com

Cover Design: Christian Ophus | Emerge Publishing, LLC
Interior Design: Anita Stumbo
Cover Photo: www.DonsImages.com

Library of Congress Cataloging-in-Publication Data

BISAC Category: HEA010000 Healthy Living; HEA016000 Naturopathy

ISBN: 978-1-943127-05-4 Hardcover
ISBN: 978-1-943127-06-1 Digital

Printed in Canada.

CONTENTS

FOREWORD

WHENEVER SOMEONE ASKS my number one strategy for fat loss, they probably expect me to mention ditching gluten or eating low-sugar impact. Maybe they assume I'll talk about how burst training coupled with weight resistance becomes your metabolic Spanx to keep you lean, toned, and healthy.

Good guesses, but not even close.

People appear surprised to learn my biggest needle mover has nothing to do with diet or exercise. If you aren't getting seven to nine hours of high quality, uninterrupted sleep every night, your best efforts for weight loss and optimal health will seriously crash.

Of course diet and exercise play significant roles, but focus solely there and you overlook strategies like sleeping sufficiently, controlling stress, and developing meaningful relationships that prove equally important to becoming lean and healthy.

That all-encompassing approach underlies *The Quest for Wellness*. Beyond just engaging your physical self, authors Dr. Mark Sherwood and Dr. Michele Neil-Sherwood challenge us to embrace a truly holistic approach to become lean, energetic, and vibrantly healthy.

Their message is disarmingly simple: Being healthy needn't become a full-time effort. Instead, they provide simple but effective strategies like eating real food, transitioning into a low-sugar impact diet, getting enough sleep, giving back, and reducing stress.

In this book you'll find a valuable diet and exercise plan, but you'll also learn how things like keeping the right mindset and connecting deeply with others foster wellness at a whole different level.

Spirituality plays a crucial role within this well-rounded approach. Science has always been a little uneasy with prayer and other spiritual approaches, occasionally dismissing it as, well, unscientific or unsubstantiated.

On the contrary, numerous studies confirm praying and positive thinking dramatically impact everything from cancer to rheumatoid arthritis to depression.

I witnessed that healing power firsthand when a hit-and-run driver struck my teenage son Grant in September 2012. While doctors appeared pessimistic, I cultivated a steadfast optimism and reached out to those closest to me for prayer, advice, and support.

During those challenging months, I learned asking for help allows others to tap into their deepest resources and serve others, which is our life purpose.

Ultimately, a combination of prayer, hope, love, and tenacity along with an amazing team of medical professionals saved Grant. He not only survived; he thrived, and today he's better than ever.

To truly care for your loved ones, you have to care for yourself first. When you aren't being your best self, you can't help others. Conversely, being a beacon of strength, resiliency, and glowing health helps other people shine their own light.

That take-control, self-empowering message runs throughout *The Quest for Wellness*. "You must want to have more energy and strength," the authors write. "And, you must want to do the simple things necessary for gaining more energy and strength ... and do these things consistently and persistently."

Steady, sustained effort pays off. While indeed simple, the strategies within these pages put you in the driver's seat of health to deliver powerful, transformative, lasting changes.

Here's to embracing your health on every level!

JJ Virgin
New York Times Best-Selling Author
The Virgin Diet
Sugar Impact Diet

INTRODUCTION

I N A WORLD WHERE HEALTHCARE costs are one of the top five expenses for any company, the only way to successfully manage the health and well-being of your workforce is through a well structured and implemented Wellness program.

Several years ago I had the good fortune to be introduced to Mark Sherwood. As a business consultant, I was seeking a professional who had deep expertise in designing and implementing a world-class Wellness program for both small and large companies. Mark's unique and effective holistic methodology gets proven results with sustainable impact.

Not only does Mark have a strong passion for wellness, fitness and balance, his expertise, experience and credentials provide the perfect foundation for *The Quest For Wellness*. His three phase approach is easy to follow and inspires the reader to stay with the program through his inspirational style.

While many approaches focus on a short-term plan to get to a specific goal, *The Quest For Wellness* takes you on a journey of self-awareness and incremental growth to equip you with a plan for life.

Mark not only coaches others to find their best self, he is a role-model for everything he professes. By purchasing *The Quest For Wellness*, you have taken the first step in changing your lifestyle to provide you with increased energy and strength in every aspect of your life.

Teri Aulph
Teri Aulph Consulting

The public has an insatiable appetite for books and products that have to do with health and wellness. The market responds to that thirst with thousands of items coming out every year and much of what the public is given are untruths, schemes and false promises, so the search continues ad nauseum. That was until Dr. Mark and Dr. Michele wrote "The Quest for Wellness." For anyone wanting true health, longevity and a life changed forever, the search is now over. Whether your wellness efforts include physical, emotional, intellectual or spiritual, you have found what you need. Take it from someone who has spent half a lifetime searching for the answer. Your answer is here and it is time to really live the rest of your life.

Major Travis Yates, Tulsa Police Department
Law Officer Magazine International Trainer of the Year

1

WHY I AM CONFIDENT
I CAN HELP YOU

I AM ONE HUNDRED PERCENT confident that I can help you gain more energy and strength.

The operative word in that statement, however, is this: *CAN*. I know that the information in this book, when applied, *can* cause you to experience more energy and strength. I have experienced this in my life and have seen it in the lives of literally hundreds of clients through the years.

There is only one thing that stands in the way of what will help you, and receiving that help. It is your will. You must *want* to have more energy and strength. And, you must *want* to do the simple things necessary for gaining more energy and strength … and do these things consistently and persistently.

When many people hear me make the previous seven sentences, they immediately put up a wall of subtle resistance, saying to themselves, "Not *me*. Whatever Mark is advocating won't work for *me*. I'd like more energy and I'd like to be stronger, but that isn't gonna happen for *me*."

Some people believe they have already tried and failed to have more energy and strength. In truth, most who *think* they have tried … haven't. Not really.

Some people believe that there is only so much energy and strength a person can experience and that this is an exhaustible supply that can be depleted and never replenished. They are wrong.

Some people believe that it is too difficult to gain more energy and strength—that it takes too many hours, too much effort, or costs too much money. Again, they are wrong on all counts.

At the same time, most of those people who don't believe they *can* have more energy and strength, secretly would *like* to be more energetic and feel stronger. They want to be able to leap out of bed in the morning, make it all the way through a variety of chores in a day, and still have a little reserve of energy as they climb into bed at night. They want to be able to play with their children or grandchildren, do their work without pain medications or flexibility limitations, and feel a basic vibrancy about their personal lives and relationships.

In other words, they have a desire for more energy and strength. They just don't think it is *possible*—not at their current age, not at their current stage of health, and not today or in the near future.

I disagree *one hundred percent*, and I want you to believe ONE MORE TIME that an increase in energy and strength just *might* be possible for YOU.

Three Things I Believe about You

There are three things I believe about you, and for you. I challenge you to believe these things about yourself.

MY BELIEF IN YOU #1: You can lead YOU

In other words, you can take charge of your own health *to a very great extent*. Physicians and medical scientists can help you with information, techniques, and from time to time, important strategies, procedures, surgeries, or medicines. But *for the most part*, your health lies within the domain of things you can do for yourself.

YOU are the one who determines what you eat and drink … what you choose to do with your time and talent … who you choose to associate with … what you choose to think, feel, and believe … and how you want to structure your particular environment both at work and at home. You are the foremost leader of *you*.

Let me repeat that statement as I invite you to memorize it:

You are the foremost leader of you.

If not you, then who? Are you blaming a spouse for any limitations, weaknesses, or negative conditions in your life? Are you blaming an employer ... the government ... your past teachers or coaches ... your childhood upbringing ... your peer group?

REALLY? Since when did you turn over all influence and controls to people who are limiting you and holding you back from your potential? And why?

Since when did you stop believing that you can do more ... fly higher ... achieve new goals ... gain more of all life's best blessings ... or experience a deeper relationship with God, other people, and your close family members? And why?

Since when did you decide to sit back and watch life go by ... sink into the coma pit you call your sofa and veg out vicariously on so-called "reality" shows rather than live your own reality ... or adopt the prevailing cultural view that there's only so much success and achievement possible and you have been left out of the mix? And *why?*

The truth is, there *is* no defined criterion for a limitation on energy and strength— at least no limitation that you are likely to reach in the next one hundred years of extreme activity! There is no fixed supply of energy meted out to a person at their birth, or after they cross an imaginary middle-age mark. There is no predetermined conclusion regarding your health. No matter what your genome might indicate as "potential" for ailments, researchers will still tell you that more than eighty percent of all negative health conditions are far more a matter of a person's lifestyle than their genetic predisposition!

You have the privilege of *deciding* that you are going to pursue more energy and strength.

You have the responsibility for determining how much more energy and strength you want to have.

You have the prerogative to choose whether you are willing to lead yourself, and HOW you want to LEAD YOURSELF.

Leading Beyond Yourself. Most people not only lead themselves. They also lead others. Parents lead their children, and sometimes middle-aged children lead their elderly parents. Teachers lead students, coaches lead teams, and employers lead employees. Those who are pastors, priests, or rabbis; doctors of all types; and people who are at the "head" of an agency, department, factory line, nonprofit group, ministry outreach, or social club also are leaders.

Leadership is of two general types: role-modeling and direct command. Role-modeling involves *showing* others an expected behavior or protocol through living example. Direct command means telling others "what to do" and usually when, how often, where, with whom, and how "to do" it. Direct command and role-modeling may have elements of "why" in the explanations given to those who follow. In many cases, both types of leadership include large amounts of *influence* that go beyond verbalizing a rule or command. Also in many cases, *both* role-modeling and direct command are involved, often simultaneously.

Why is it important to recognize this beyond-you form of leadership? Because if you are part of a group of any kind, you likely want that group to *succeed*. And the success of your group is going to be in direct proportion to the overall energy and strength level of all the members of the group combined. Think about this for a moment: if you have ten people in a group and they are functioning at different energy and strength levels, you can "add" up those levels for a total of some type. Let's say your people or family members are functioning at levels 9, 8, 7, 7, 5, 4, 3, 3, 2, 2. That total is going to be 50. That's fifty, by the way, of a total possible 100 points. Let's say another ten-person group—perhaps a rival team or rival company group—is functioning at an energy and strength level of 9, 8, 8, 8, 7, 7, 7, 6, 5, 4. It is not only significant that nobody in this second group is functioning below level "four" but the sum reveals a total of 69 points. That's a nearly twenty percent HIGHER level of functioning than group one!

The higher a group is in "energy," the more that group is likely to communicate more frequently (all members communicating with all members), be more creative, produce more work per time unit (be it hour, week, month, or quarter), to seek and acquire more information (including information about competitors, new research related to a product line, or new methods for greater efficiency or productivity), have higher morale, have fewer sick days per year as a group, and be more responsive to customers, vendors, and other departments or groups that may be encountered.

The higher a group is in "strength," the more the group will be able to sustain its efforts, the more willing it will be to work overtime, and the more likely the group will be to seek to build "permanence" and "ongoing stability" into any project or product.

In the real world, greater energy and greater strength means more innovation and marketplace appeal for the group, greater brand recognition, and greater financial success. In the world of families, it likely means stronger familial bonds. In the world of religious groups, it likely means a stronger "witness" or appeal to new members. In the world of health care, it can mean more satisfied patients with more successful procedures and a more positive "health profile" for a patient load. And so on.

There are hundreds of corporate and organizational profiles you can consult that will verify these results. When you think "Silicon Valley" do you think high energy and high strength, or low energy and low strength? The same could be asked for the upper northwest, where Microsoft and dozens of other high-tech companies have their headquarters.

When you think of successful military campaigns, do you see greater positive results for those with high-energy and high-strength methods and personnel, or low-energy and low-strength methods and personnel?

When you think of school systems or sports teams, do you see better "scores" for those marked by high energy and high strength, or low energy and low strength?

Again, high nearly always comes out ahead of low, except perhaps in environments we might call convents, monasteries, spas, or beach resorts ... but there, the very purpose of the group is likely to BE low energy at the consumer or participant level, even if it is not the purpose in the corporate office or upper echelons of leadership in those places.

What about you personally?

Do you want to be part of a high-energy, high-strength *group* ... or a low-energy, low-strength group? The vast majority of people will vote "high" every time.

If you are the *leader* of a group, it is part of your responsibility to build greater energy and strength into the group. And that brings me back to the book you are holding in your hand.

What is good for YOU as an individual is going to be good for your group, your team, your family. And you can very likely do something to infuse the principles of this book into your group. I'll offer some suggestions along the way, but keep in mind at the outset that *all* of the principles in this book work at the communal level as well as the individual level.

MY BELIEF IN YOU #2: You can change your perspective

Most people are in a two-fold rut—like the two tracks of a vehicle in the mud. First, they are in a rut when it comes to their habits. They do the same things day after day, and rarely give much thought to why they have adopted the habits they have. In the vast majority of cases, they are reinforcing their own bad habits through repetition—they are reinforcing their own poor health.

Second, they are in a mental and emotional rut. Most people are in a rut when it comes to the way they see life. They rarely question the choices they routinely make or the emotional responses they have adopted through thousands of repetitions. They no longer see a bright future—one filled with hope, beauty, enthusiasm, or deep vitality!

Several decades ago, one of the pioneers in the nutrition world began to talk to her neighbors about basic health principles. She didn't go out seeking to talk with her neighbors. Rather, her neighbors came to her. They had seen the poor health of her children, and how her children were suddenly more healthy and energetic. They wanted to know what she had done to turn around the health level of her family. This woman told them what she had learned and what she had started doing, and then she helped them make little packets of vitamins and minerals to try in their families. The health of the entire neighborhood improved!

This woman was not medically trained and she knew that she could get in trouble for practicing medicine without a license, so she said this to those who came to her for advice: "I am not a doctor and I cannot diagnose your ailments or prescribe medicines for you. But I do know this. When you tell me how you are feeling, I know that healthy people don't feel that way! When you tell me what 'ails you,' I know that healthy people don't have those ailments. So, my suggestion is that you do what will take you toward a goal of better health. Do the healthful things. Don't focus on your ailments, pains, or 'conditions.' Focus on the goal of better health in your body, mind, emotions, and spirit."

I echo her advice: GO FOR A NEW GOAL!

In a nutshell, that is the perspective of this book. Set yourself in the direction of MORE ENERGY and MORE STRENGTH. Don't focus on your limitations or past experiences. Focus instead on a new goal!

Let me be very quick to say to you that I am in no way asking you to stop taking a particular medication or following a specific health protocol prescribed for you by a reputable physician. What I am asking you to do is to change your perspective about yourself and to stop thinking about yourself as a sick person— and instead, see yourself as a person who is in hot pursuit of becoming a healthy person! Again, here's a good statement for you to memorize:

I am a committed person in pursuit of greater health—more energy and more strength!

No matter your current level of energy and strength, you can have *more* energy and strength.

Rather than say, "I have arthritis"—change your perspective. Say, "I am going to pursue a life without joint pain. I am going to do what I can to have greater flexibility, range of motion, and renewed cartilage."

Rather than say, "I am a diabetic"—change your perspective. Say, "I am going to pursue a life in which my weight is under control and what I eat is in the right quantities of the right foods eaten at the right times."

Rather than say, "I have high blood pressure"—change your perspective. Say, "I am going to do the right things to control my stress levels, improve the cardiovascular health of my heart and blood vessels, and bring maximum oxygen and nutrients to every cell of my body."

The words don't change physical conditions—but the pursuit of new habits and a new lifestyle *will* change physical conditions.

Am I promising you a full cure for a dire disease or a debilitating condition? No ... but I am promising you that if you will pursue new HEALTH and WHOLENESS goals, you can have *BETTER* health than you presently have in your current state.

For most people, a ten-percent improvement in overall energy and strength is not only noticeable, but thoroughly appreciated. A twenty-percent improvement in energy and strength is going to be fantastic! A thirty- or forty-percent improvement is going to put the person into the stratosphere of ecstasy! And anything beyond that is going to leave them wondering why they never lived the way that led to such dramatic improvement of their overall life!

MY BELIEF IN YOU #3: You can be more WHOLE

Every person is a *whole* entity that encompasses far more than the body. You know that. But have you truly *considered* what that means?

Every human being lives simultaneously in four dimensions:

1. *The Physical.* This includes the dimension of their physical body and also the physical world around their body—their "environment" or "space" that provides the physical context for their gaining of nutrients and expelling waste.

2. *The Emotional.* This includes the broad realm of feelings and responses to both internal stimuli and external stimuli. It especially includes the realm of relationships.

3. *The Intellectual.* This includes the dimension of ideas and creativity. It includes a person's rationality and ability to make sound choices. It includes the person's sense of productivity, their understanding of efficiency, and their baseline definitions for quality performance.

4. *The Spiritual.* This includes the foundation of a person's values and beliefs. It includes their understanding about their Creator and what it means to be in relationship with their Creator.

In western civilization, far more than eastern civilizations, we tend to divide these aspects of human existence, primarily for the purposes of study and evaluation, but in truth, there are no clear-cut divisions in one human being or in human beings collectively. We are recognizing increasingly in science and in general cultural philosophy that we cannot *divide* a person and we especially cannot separate physical well-being from a person's emotional, mental, and spiritual well-being. We exist as an entity that has different facets, but these facets are interrelated and cannot be separated in any kind of real way. In theory, perhaps, but never in application.

This leads to an understanding, of course, that all aspects of a human's existence are intended to be lived out in harmony—fully integrated and functioning *as a whole.* Each facet of life impacts all other facets. And the goal is to achieve a balance among all facets.

Health is not simply a matter of *physical* health. A person cannot be truly *healthy* unless he or she is healthy in emotions, intellect, and spirit.

In the same way, it is impossible for a person to have extremely high energy or strength physically without also having energy and strength emotionally, mentally, and spiritually. Any athlete who competes at the top international levels knows this. Winning the medal or winning the game is very often a mental, emotional, and yes, even a spiritual endeavor as much as it is a matter of physical coordination, skill, and training.

Not long ago I heard a sports commentator conclude that a particular team had won the "big game" because "the team wanted the win more than its opponents wanted it." The *will* to win—something that might be envisioned as a combination of spiritual desire and emotional ambition—is a powerful force. So, too, is the *will* to live … and the *will* to reach a goal … and the *will* to complete a task … and the *will* to maintain one's core values through extreme difficulty.

My contention is that no person is going to become *whole* without a concerted, focused *will* to become whole. The integration of the human self does not happen by accident. It doesn't happen without intention. A person must aim for wholeness and pursue it with a concentration of willpower.

Yes, you *can* lead your own life and choose to change.

Yes, you *can* change the way you perceive life and seek to go for a new goal.

Yes, you *can* begin to see your life as a whole entity requiring an integration of all facets of your being.

And at the heart of all this is the concept of BALANCE.

Each aspect of human life must be pursued in balance with all other facets. Only then is wholeness going to be attainable and sustainable.

Can it be done? Yes.

Is it extremely difficult? No.

Does it require a choice? Yes.

My challenge to you is this:

Lead a lockstep life. Pursue wholeness
with a balanced approach.

The rest of this book is devoted to telling you *how*, and seeking to motivate you to do it!

2

THE PURSUIT OF WHOLENESS

WHAT IS WELLNESS? How do *you* define it?

For the purposes of this book, wellness goes beyond the general cultural definition of "absence of illness." Lots of people live without a definable disease, but many of those people will readily tell you that they don't feel all that good much of the time. The terms "physically fit" and "thin" also should not be confused with wellness. There are many people who are thin or who work out several times a week who do not manifest wellness.

In this book, wellness refers to being:

- *Spiritually connected to God and to other people.* It is focused on a relationship that involves a person's innermost being. Spiritual wellness has very little to do with being religious (the keeping of specified man-generated rituals) or belonging to a particular religious group.

- *Intellectually stimulated.* Wellness is associated with displaying ongoing curiosity and ongoing learning, with a disciplined approach to the study of, and reflection upon, new information as well as old information.

- *Emotionally balanced*—with the other side of the balance bar being "reason." How a person feels and how a person *thinks* need to be in sync. This keeps the person from uncontrolled emotions that can hinder relationships, jobs, and the performance of even basic tasks. A "well" person does not severely stifle, dismiss, or deny emotions, but rather, is aware of his or her emotions and seeks to use the energy from emotions for productive purposes.

- *Physically strong and energized* in order to accomplish the basic goals that the person believes he *should* accomplish in a given day or other time span. Physical health becomes a balance of input and output—what a person takes into the body (food, beverages, air) and what a person releases from the body (in the form of work, exercise, and other forms of calorie expenditure, as well as physical elimination of waste—primarily from the digestive tract, skin, and lungs).

Furthermore, these four areas need to function in sync—they are intertwined and feed on one another. When a person is active physically, he tends to feel better emotionally. When a person feels better, he usually finds it is easier to learn, remember, and synthesize information. When a person is functioning in wellness, he is more attuned to spiritual needs and opportunities for spiritual growth.

Every person was designed by our Creator for WELLNESS. God made us as whole individuals and desires for us to be whole. The fact that most of us do *not* live that way is a fact that *CAN* be remedied!

Wellness Is Learned ... and Is Subject to *Practice*

We do not automatically acquire wellness. We must learn and apply its principles.

What we learn, we learn through repeated exposure to concepts, and that implies *practice*. We rehearse what we practice in our memory, and we practice what we learn mostly through application of information to real-life situations. All of that should be very encouraging to you. Even if you have learned faulty information about health and wellness, and even if you have applied that information in negative ways, you can *relearn* good wellness principles and also learn how to apply and practice them in beneficial ways!

Practice Makes Perfect. The old saying "practice makes perfect" is mostly true. Unless, of course, a person is practicing the wrong behaviors or doing them incorrectly! Repeated activities produce habits. In an exercise setting, "repetitions" are a part of strength building. In a spiritual setting, repeated activities are often associated with spiritual disciplines. In the realm of intellect and learning, repetition is the way we learned our multiplication tables (or how to use a calculator), the alphabet, and a wide variety of definitions that are unconsciously folded into daily life. We tend to brush our teeth because of early-childhood repeated patterns, and whether we admit it or not, most of us hold to opinions and beliefs we learned early in life as a result of daily or frequent reinforcement related to "do this" and "don't do that" admonitions from the adults who were responsible for our childhood training.

Once a person has acquired a habit, it is often difficult to change a habit ... but it can be done. It takes intention (meaning to do it), focus and consistency (regularly doing the new habit in a correct way, time, or frequency), and rewards (for making the change).

If you are willing to embark on a path to greater WELLNESS, you need to recognize that:

- There are some thing things you need to *choose to change* in your habits. You may know what some of those are, and may already be groaning about the change you know would be "good" for you.
- You are going to be faced with the challenge of becoming consistent and focused. Change doesn't happen haphazardly. It doesn't happen by hoping or wishing for something "vaguely like" an ideal that you desire.

- You are going to need to find ways of motivating yourself to make and sustain the change, and that usually means finding rewards that are pleasurable and meaningful to you and others around you for goals reached as you make your way to greater wholeness. There's more on this later but for now, recognize that you likely need to come up with *new* ways of rewarding your own good behavior and new healthful habits—you can't reward a weight loss goal with a hot fudge sundae, or reward your attendance at a Sunday morning worship service with a next-Saturday evening excursion to a strip club. Rewards need to be in line with the overall concept of wellness—what is GOOD for a person in one area needs to be GOOD for the person in all areas of life, and that also includes being GOOD for others who share your common life (especially family members).

Practice Takes Time. Practice is also a concept that translates into time.

I once was asked, "How much time do you spend maintaining your health?"

I replied, "I'm not a good person to ask."

The reason for my reply is that for several decades now, I have spent *way* more time exercising and body building than most people have, are, will, or *can* spend. In part, I did this because it was my *job*. In high school, I worked out in order to succeed in sports and get a college scholarship. In college, I worked hard physically to be the best I could be in my field of sports, and to prepare for a pro career. When I went to Australia to play pro ball, I worked out physically to stay strong and hope for a pro contract back in the United States. And on and on it went. I worked for many years as a police officer and I was very committed all through those years to being at the top of my physical ability in order to do my job with the greatest degree of excellence.

What I know is this … it does take time to live in wellness.

And I know that it doesn't take nearly as much time as many people think.

Give yourselves ninety minutes a day devoted to *your* personal wellness.

Does that seem like a lot of time to you?

There's a high probability that you are already spending ninety minutes a day in ways that are contributing to a *lack* of wellness. Most American adults spend at least that amount of time a day sitting on a sofa watching rather mindless television or playing computer games or surfing the internet for information that isn't vital to their job performance. Most Americans "squander" their drive time—they don't listen to information that might be informative or motivational, or spiritually uplifting. Many Americans actually spend as much time in drive-through lanes purchasing fast food that isn't good for their bodies as they would need to spend cooking a simple meal of whole foods that *are* nutritionally beneficial.

In the pages that follow, I'm going to recommend certain

activities that can be done *concurrently.* This does not mean double-tasking, which, for the most part, has been shown to be counterproductive to both quality of performance and enjoyment. "Concurrent" in this book means to do something within the same twenty-four- or forty-eight-hour period.

Let's break it down for an example:

- **Physical:** sustained physical activity a day
  Activity, such as walking. . . . . 10 minutes
  Taking time to prepare and eat
        two vegetables a day. . . . . 10 minutes
  Go to bed earlier for increased sleep . . . . 30 minutes

- **Emotional:** Write in a personal journal . . . . . 10 minutes

- **Intellectual:** Take a daily "mini" vacation
  In world of your imagination . . . . 5 minutes
  Read a nonfiction book (or manual). . . . . . . 10 minutes

- **Spiritual:** Sit in silence. . . . . 5 minutes
  Read the Bible or other spiritual material . . . 10 minutes

90 minutes!

Which part of that *can't* you do? Try trading out journal-writing time for media time. Perhaps listen to a nonfiction CD on your way to and from work, or listen to the Bible in a recorded format. Use part of your noon hour at work to lace on your walking shoes and go for a walk.

If you only spend 9 minutes a day exercising one day, go for

11 minutes the next. Don't beat yourself up if you don't get to bed a half hour earlier than usual. Consider why you didn't and evaluate adjustments you might make for the next evening. If you can write everything you want to say in your journal in 3 minutes, so be it. There are no "must do's" in this program when it comes to time commitment, only "good to do's."

Never lose sight of the fact that you are blessed to have a mind that is capable of making sound decisions, and a body that is capable of functioning relatively efficiently, and that you likely are already living in a degree of wellness. Now is the time to give *yourself* the gift of a little more focus and time to make your *total wellness* a priority.

A Mental Adjustment. As important as a time commitment to change is a commitment to a change in the way you currently THINK.

This book presents a way to take on the thinking habits that probably got you into the state you are presently in—a "lack" of wellness.

The mental adjustment means thinking *differently* and also *making different choices.*

Are you willing to exchange a sugary dessert for a whole piece of ripe fruit? Are you willing to accept that your body truly *needs* more water and more sleep?

Are you willing to address your personal stress level, which nearly always correlates directly with food intake, emotional distress, and relationship difficulties? Are you willing to evaluate all of your current responsibilities to see what might be lessened or eliminated as a means of controlling stress?

Are you willing to stop trying to be everything, to everybody, all the time, with perfection as the only standard of performance? Are you willing to give up double-tasking?

Are you willing to change your *concept* of mid-morning and mid-afternoon snacks to produce more sustained energy and fewer sugar highs or sugar lows?

Are you willing to develop your spiritual life and to get involved with people who share your beliefs and who can help you reinforce your spiritual goals?

These are all DECISIONS and CHOICES that are at the heart of genuine life change. And … they all relate to wellness. If you don't recognize that at this point, are you willing to accept the *possibility* of this being true?

Bravery for a New World. Many of us have read in our past the book that described a "Brave New World." For some, a quest for wellness becomes the "new world" that will truly require a degree of courage on their part. Part of the reason for this is that we don't live in the world of our childhood. I realize that you *know* that, but have you truly pondered that fact?

The food of today does not have the nutrients in it that food once had. Modern packaging and processing techniques have stripped many foods of their nutritional value, and in many parts of our nation, soils have been depleted of the minerals that once made their way into home-grown foods.

The pace of today is not as slow as it once was. A woman recently lamented to me, "I don't know how my mother did it. She cooked three meals a day, kept the books for my father's business, drove my sister and me to school every day and picked us up, attended all of our recitals and games, and took us to art lessons. She ran a smooth-functioning home that was clean and orderly, and I have no memories of stacks of laundry ready to be washed or folded. What am I doing wrong?"

We talked about this a little and came to a couple of insights: Her mother did not feel the need to stay connected to social media, soap operas, or news programs for several hours a day … her mother could run all of her shopping and appointment errands within a four-mile radius of their home … her mother grew flowers in her garden (which meant she never needed to stop at a floral shop) and vegetables in the backyard plot … her mother was able to pick oranges and peaches from backyard trees … the school was only six blocks from home … and her mother often used her time spent sitting by the YWCA pool while her daughters took swimming lessons as an opportunity for catching up on magazine reading. The television set was mostly off during her childhood. There was only one phone shared by the four people in the household. There was no constant concern with social media or the use of multiple "apps" to tell her mother what to do or when. Yes … she had a simpler life, but it was no less productive, and no less rewarding. Some of us need to rethink.

It does take bravery *not* to follow the cultural pressure to stay connected with everybody all of the time. It does take bravery *not* to care whether you see or know or do the latest and newest or most popular thing. It does take bravery to want to be *well* in every area of your life rather than *just get by.*

The best changes are ones that are made gradually … but nevertheless *are made.* Step by step. Day by day.

Choose to ignore the media hype.
Avoid the fads. Take intentional, consistent,
daily steps on a firm foundation!

Are you ready to launch into a brave new way of living a life on a path to genuine WELLNESS? Then read on … .

3

THREE IMPORTANT KEYS
TO WELLNESS SUCCESS

A<small>T THE VERY OUTSET</small> of our discussion about wellness, let me
address three very important keys that I know, from years
of experience, are vital to your experiencing success with
a Wellness Plan. These keys are:

1. The Setting of Goals
2. The Keeping of a Personal Journal
3. Periodically Synthesizing Information and Establishing
   Balance before moving on to higher levels of understanding or practice

1. The Value of Setting Goals

There's a question among the old-timers in my area that I've
always enjoyed: "Are you going somewhere or are you just
traveling?"

Many people are rather mindless wanderers through life. They "go with the flow," rarely stopping to question why they are doing what they are doing.

Now, I'm all in favor of taking time for leisurely walks to enjoy nature, including time to stop and smell the flowers along the way. But as an overall plan for life, there's not a lot of value in simply going with the flow and ending up at the bottom of a large drainage reservoir!

As a whole, our culture isn't going where I want to end up. I don't want to end up in a nursing facility with someone else making the most important decisions about my life for me. I don't want to end up impoverished—in any dimension of life. I don't want to end up without good friendships and loving relationships twenty years from now. I don't want to waste the time God has given me in unimportant or even negative activities. I don't want to pollute my body or lungs with chemicals that can kill me if they are taken in excess, and who knows just how much it takes to cross over into excess?

I'm not into the latest dance craze or clubbing or playing poker with a scotch in one hand and a cigar in my mouth. I'm not into spending ten hours a week watching prime-time television programs that nearly always have an illicit sexual affair, a murder, or violence as a vital part of the plot line.

No, I do NOT want to end up where the culture will take me if I choose NOT to exert any will of my own to develop a different way of life.

When we each take a look at our life and decide how we want

to live, we invariably are setting goals—perhaps short-term and perhaps long-term.

One of the best approaches I know is to take the VERY long-term goal-setting approach. Where do you want to end up AFTER you die? What kind of life do you envision you will have THEN? And what will it take for you to have a high level of assurance that you are going to be able to attain that type of life?

Equally important, in my opinion, are the goals you have for the life you want to be living just hours before you die!

I once saw a cartoon in which a doctor was writing out a prescription for a slightly overweight patient. The doctor said, "Would you rather I write a prescription for exercise one hour a day, or one that called for you to contact an undertaker and keep him on a twenty-four-hour notice?"

This seemed a bit harsh to me, but the more I reflected on this, the more I realized that millions of people in our world are *driven* to succeed, but rarely do they consider that all the success they desire will not matter if they are dead. The things we truly value in life, and increasingly so as we age, are our health, our peace of mind, and our loving relationships with family members and friends. Money, career success, and possessions don't really matter if there's no health to enjoy them, no loved ones to enjoy them with, and peace of mind that includes peace with God.

Most people WANT to have love, health, and spiritual peace as they face their final years, months, days, or hours. Those are good goals to pursue *now*.

The Ultimate Goal: Being the Best YOU Can Be. A serious approach to goal setting is likely going to end up with you answering the question: What is the Best YOU that you desire to become? All of my personal goals are within the context of my desire to be the best person I can be—not only for the sake of those I love and others who watch my life, but also so that I can give the greatest honor to my Creator.

In making your goals, I suggest that you start with character and reputation issues *first*, and then work backwards. Ask God who HE wants you to be and what He desires for you to accomplish in your life, and that will give you a good start in defining HOW you want to live.

I have no desire to set a goal that God does not desire for me to attain. To do so would be folly, in my opinion. I see little chance of success without God's assistance. I also know that if I attain a goal that God has not authorized for me, it will fall far short of my definition of "treasure." It will have little long-term satisfaction and virtually no eternal meaning.

As you set goals, I encourage you to pray about them *in advance*. Give serious thought to what you believe is totally within your ultimate purpose for being on this earth. What is in alignment with the talents you have been given from birth, and the skills you have been led to develop through the years. What brings you the deepest pleasure and fulfillment in your life? It is in this rich soil of fulfillment and giftedness that your goals should be planted.

Realistic and Attainable. I personally choose to set goals that have a built-in degree of guilt-free SUCCESS. I want to have goals that are achievable and failure-proof.

As you set goals:

1. **Be Realistic.** Realistic nearly always translates into "achievable." If you cannot envision yourself actually REACHING a goal, it isn't a realistic one for you.

2. **Short Term and Long Term.** As you set goals, make sure to include goals that are short term, perhaps three months out. Even that may be too long a time period for you. If you find it a little overwhelming to think in terms of "next season" or "next year," try setting goals for the NEXT TWO WEEKS. If you can do something and achieve something for two weeks, you will have PROOF that you can do it for two more!

3. **Establish Time Allotments.** Some people find it easier to set goals if they are mapping out the time required for pursuing a goal. For example, rather than think of walking daily, a person may find it easier to commit to ten minutes a day, walking in a neighborhood park. It may be easier for you to think of two thirty-minute exercise times in a week rather than ten minutes a day. The weekly total is far more important than the daily amount.

4. **Consult with Others.** I recommend you check your goals with a personal trainer, or perhaps your physician,

or someone who functions in your life as an accountability partner. An accountability partner is a person who has your best interests at heart, who will listen to you and give you their honest feedback, and who will expect you periodically to give an update of your progress. Discuss with your trainer or accountability partner what you are going to do to reach your goals (not just the end result but the PROCESS you intend to follow in pursuit of the goal), and also *why* you have set the goals you have written down. Sometimes a person with an objective viewpoint can see strengths or flaws in your goals that you cannot see clearly.

5. **Become Committed to Your Goals.** Come into agreement with your trainer, counselor, or an accountability partner that you WILL do what you have set for yourself as a goal. Set deadlines for checking in to give a progress report.

6. **Revisit Your Goals Weekly.** Reminding yourself of your goals is a way to stay on track, and to remain motivated.

7. **Make a Decision to Endure.** Decide within yourself that, if you do NOT reach a specific goal in a desired time frame, you will continue to pursue your goal and you will REFUSE to become discouraged.

8. **Revise if Necessary.** If you have prolonged difficulty in sticking to the PROCESS you designed for pursuing a

goal, talk with your trainer, counselor, or accountability partner about ways in which you may need to revise your goal or the process you planned. You may have set a goal that is too high, or set an implementation plan that is too ambitious given your other time commitments.

Turning Your Goals into a Plan. A plan sets goals into time and space. It is a road map, of sorts, about what you intend to do, when, where, and sometimes with whom.

A plan takes you from where you are today (Point A) to where you want to be (Point B), likely with a number of checkpoints along the way (Point A1, A2, A3, and so forth).

As you map out your plan, make sure it:

- *Is Balanced.* The plan should include all four areas related to wellness.

- *Has Periodic Checkpoints for Analysis.* You need to take stock occasionally to make sure you are still on track.

- *Is Rewarding.* All of the rewards do not come at the end of achieving a goal. Most of them should come *as you make your journey toward a goal.*

A person once described a trip he and his family had taken. They had originally planned to take an entire week to go from Point A in Dallas to Point B in Seattle. They planned to stay a week in Seattle, and then take another route home that would also take an entire week. Those three weeks were part of their "plan," but the plan also included an option—the man had taken a full month off from work, as had his wife, and they knew they *could* spend as much as thirty days on this particular adventure.

Fast forwarding to the end of their story …

They never did make it to Seattle. They had too much fun exploring back roads through New Mexico and Colorado before taking on the California mountains and finally the California coastline. They meandered their way through Arizona and back to Texas. Some entire days they spent lying on a beach or hiking a mountain trail. They stopped to ride ponies one day, watched a horse show another day, took a cable car all over San Francisco on yet another day, and attended a major league ball game in Los Angeles.

They considered it the trip of their lifetime as a family! This man told me they laughed more and talked more seriously about countless topics than they ever had as a family. They did things they all mutually enjoyed. And they left behind all concerns about world news, as well as all emails. They did allow themselves fifteen minutes each late afternoon for what they called a "blitz" of messages posted on social media, in part to document for themselves the visual images of their trip.

Did they have a goal? Yes. The goal was "HAVE A GOOD VACATION WITH THE FAMILY." The plan had called for a trip north and west, and they did go west, and to a degree, north. The plan had called for 3-4 weeks and they did that. They did not follow the route they had initially planned to take, but

in many ways, that is true for most people who make plans—
there always seem to be changes that are wise to make along the
way. The overall plan, however, had been to travel by car to see
new things and have new experiences, and therefore make new
and good memories as a family. The plan worked! Their goal was
achieved.

And the bottom line is this: if a plan is altered and you still
achieve the goal you set, that's the BETTER plan.

Don't be afraid to take detours if they are good ones. Just
don't lose sight of the ultimate goal.

Goals and plans tend to intersect in this way:

Make Goals, Develop a Plan for Achieving Them,
and then Make a Goal to Work the Plan!

2. The Value of Maintaining a Personal Journal

A journal is a place for documenting your journey toward Wellness, and also recording your own personal insights, emotions,
and progress along the way. It is a place for jotting down creative
ideas, putting words to your innermost dreams and desires, and
capturing spiritual insights that sometimes seem fleeting. It is
also a place for keeping track of very practical data.

Above all, a personal journal is just that: PERSONAL. You
are invited as part of your Wellness Plan to keep a personal journal and to use it in various ways. How you structure this journal,
when you write in it, how often you write in it, how *much* you
write in it, and what you eventually do with it is *your* business.

Be cautious in letting others read your journal. Not all that you write in your journal is refined or should be published.

Your personal journal is a place to note the progress you make in a weight-loss program (if one is necessary for you), your fitness program, your emotions, your innovative ideas, your spiritual discernments, and your concerns.

What is the value to you?

You will have a document that you can review periodically. In nearly all cases, people who reflect on their own journals find themselves grateful for the progress they are making in life and also find themselves motivated to continue the process.

You will not have to resort to "memory" to recall moments of your own brilliance or achievement. The journal acts as a lasting memory device. This frees many people to be more spontaneous in their approach to life (think "freer" and often more "authentic") … they have more mental and emotional energy to give to others and to use in impacting their personal world.

The journal also becomes something of a "visionary" statement about your life—it reflects the person you believe you are destined to become, and the purpose for your life as you understand it. We tend to become what we say we will do and who we say that we are. A journal is a good place to record those self-declarations.

3. The Value of Synthesizing Information and Gaining Balance

This Wellness Plan calls for you to take on four dimensions of change simultaneously. It calls for you to develop physical health (energy and strength), emotional well-being, intellectual vibrancy, and spiritual depth. It invites you to do so in a fairly coordinated manner over three phases.

At two points you are invited to sit back and reflect on your own progress and to make certain that each area of your life is in sync with all other areas of your life.

The best approach is to make certain that you have mastered all of the behaviors in each dimension before moving on to the next level.

Synergy is a wonderful concept—by definition, it is when two or more parts of something work together to create an impact that is greater than the additive sum of the individual parts.

Although you will be pursuing the four dimensions of life somewhat separately, the greater truth is that you are a *whole* person. What happens in one area of your life impacts all other areas. The Wellness Plan calls for you to recognize that phenomenon and embrace it as a gift of God to you.

When spirit, mind, emotions, and body are working *together*, a release of joy, energy, and renewed strength is nearly always the result!

4

First Steps First
Phase 1

As STATED in the previous chapter, the Wellness Plan in this book calls for a person to address four areas of life concurrently and in harmony. These dimensions of life are:

PHYSICAL — EMOTIONAL — INTELLECTUAL — SPIRITUAL

Imagine four people walking with their arms linked down a path that is wide enough for all four of them to move easily. They are *striding* together, probably in step with one another. But choose to see them as doing so with shoulders back, chins up, and a big smile on their faces. There's joy in their walk, not drudgery. They are not soldiers, but highly compatible "friends" on a walk that is purposeful and fulfilling. That's the picture I want YOU to have in your mind about YOUR journey to wellness.

49

The process is divided into three phases—first steps, next steps, and ongoing steps.

First Steps First. Every journey begins with a single step. There's always a "start point." That's true for the journey to wellness. Below, you will find the items suggested as "FIRST STEPS" in

---

FIRST STEPS —

PHYSICAL

- Move more
- Do 10 minutes of walking or other activity 5 times a week
- Eliminate all sugar-based drinks or snacks
- Add 2 vegetables to every day
- Know your "baseline" numbers (weight, BMI, cholesterol, blood pressure, heart rate)
- Eat a piece of fresh fruit as your dessert
- Increase your water intake
- Get sufficient sleep

EMOTIONAL

Identify your stressors:

- Financial
- "Control" issues
- Conflict/Anger issues
- Monitor your self-talk
- Evaluate the spectrum of your responsibilities and commitments
- Identify someone to hold you accountable
- Prepare yourself emotionally for wellness to require sustained effort

---

Set Goals + Consolidate and Balance + Reset Goals +

each of the four dimensions above. And following that, you'll find additional information related to most of the behaviors listed in each category.

PHASE 1

INTELLECTUAL

- Choose or start a "course" or identify a new nonfiction book to read
- Take a daily 5-minute mini vacation
- Choose to "single-task" and to FOCUS your ideas

SPIRITUAL

- Spend 5–10 minutes in silence each day
- Engage in deep breathing (6 breaths) three times a day
- Read the Bible or other deeply meaningful spiritual literature for 10 minutes
- Get involved with people who share your beliefs

Get Counseling if you need it + Keep a Personal Journal

Notes about the PHYSICAL Dimension of Phase 1

1. More movement in your day.

A simple way to add more movement in your life is to follow the 2-20 rule: Stand two minutes for every twenty minutes you sit. Get up from your desk at least once every twenty minutes and walk a little—even if just to the water cooler to fill your water bottle or to take a walk to the stairwell, climb a flight of stairs, and then return to your floor and desk.

S-t-r-e-t-c-h as you move from a sitting to standing position.

Your body was created to *move*. It feels better if you keep moving—in fact, the lymph system of your body requires physical activity in order for it to be activated! Adding more movement to your day can be as simple as:

- Parking a little further away from the front door of the store or your office
- Taking the steps instead of the elevator, even if for only a floor or two (perhaps the last two floors before the floor in which your apartment or office is located)
- Dancing with the vacuum cleaner
- Walking the golf course instead of using a cart
- Walking the dog around the neighborhood rather than simply letting the dog out into the backyard

Wearing a pedometer seems to help many people. This little device, attached to your belt or to your shoes, measures how many steps you take in a given time frame. Set yourself a goal of 10,000 steps a day.

The best approach to take is to put on your walking shoes as soon as possible after you rise in the morning. This does two things—it makes it easier for you to count the TOTAL steps you take during the day, and it sets your "mind" toward the idea that you CAN and SHOULD go for an extended walk. In many cases, people find it easier to leave their walking shoes on all day—and perhaps carry "dress" shoes to work in a briefcase or tote bag. In some cases, I have met people who have 2–3 pairs of shoes in a filing cabinet or cupboard in their office. They only wear those "dress" shoes when they are meeting with clients or customers who may not readily appreciate "gym" shoes as part of their executive-style deliberations.

> Put exercise on your calendar as an
> "appointment with self."

2. Find an exercise that you really enjoy.

I recommend walking as the easiest, least expensive, and most "doable" exercise for most people, but the key is always to do an exercise that you really enjoy.

The exercise you enjoy is the exercise you will actually DO!

Think back to your childhood. While you may not be up for climbing a tree, you may find that you'd like to get back on a bicycle or that you might enjoy finding someone with whom to shoot baskets or play tennis. You may want to try out an exercise class that puts rhythm to music (either in floor exercises or swimming pool exercises). Most team sports or competitive sports do not provide as much exercise "value" (either in aerobics or weight training) but they do add variety to your activity in a way that reintroduces PLEASURE to the idea of moving.

In addition to finding an activity you enjoy, choose to exercise in a PLACE that you find pleasurable and safe. Many cities now have well-lit walking and cycling paths, some of which extend for many miles. Many malls or shopping centers invite people to walk their hallways and sidewalks. A wide variety of gym settings are available that often have healthful eating areas for purchasing a nutritious smoothie or protein drink (making it all the easier to exercise during a lunch hour or before work).

Periodically through the months ahead, you may want to change activities or venues. The more variety you can add to your exercise, the more you are likely to stick with it over time.

If possible, find someone to walk with or go to the gym with—even if you aren't using the same machines or walking the same path at the same time. You'll be more motivated to go and have more fun if there's a social element to your exercise times.

3. Eliminate sugar from snacks and beverages.

Americans consume about 130 pounds of sugar a year. That breaks down to about 22 teaspoons daily. Roughly 67% of this consumption happens at home.

Sugar is a major contributor to the aging process. It also damages cells and promotes chronic disease.

Sugar increasingly seems to be a form of "bait" in order to elicit child cooperation, church attendance (free donuts in the hospitality area), meeting attendance (refreshments will be served), and even eating in general (just wait until you see dessert). Even in hospitals we find employees saying to patients, "Do you want red Jell-O or green?" Both are sugar loaded and *bad* for health, yet sugar-based gelatin is a mainstay on hospital menus! (Are we nuts?)

How much sugar are *you* consuming daily? *Get real.*

4. Add more veggies to your day.

The two additional servings of vegetables you add to your daily eating plan might include a handful of lettuce or raw greens laced with black pepper and a dash of lemon juice. It might be four to six ounces of steamed vegetables. There are no restrictions on the vegetables at this point, other than this: don't smother the vegetable in any kind of sauce, dressing, or fat.

The older a person becomes, the more difficult it is to maintain the basic metabolism to get the maximum benefits from the same degree of exercise that the person "used to do" when younger. We each have to do more in order to maintain metabolism.

A key to this is in increased exercise sessions over time. But a second key is nearly as effective: changing one's diet to have low-fat protein, only quality monounsaturated fats, and more high-quality carbohydrates in the form of fresh fruits and vegetables. This dietary plan helps the body rebuild, supplies a steady supply of energy, and helps avoid storing excess fat.

5. Know your baseline numbers.

If you have not been exercising regularly, see your physician for a quick check of your body. This is also the time to get the baseline numbers you'll want to have as you chart your progress to greater physical health. These baseline numbers include weight, and more importantly your BMI (body mass index number that tells you the percentage of your body that is fat), your cholesterol (both good and bad—HDL and LDL—as well as cholesterol total), blood pressure, and heart rate.

6. Have fruit for dessert.

The sugar in fruit is not the same as the sugar in a candy bar or piece of chocolate cake. The natural sugars in fruit metabolize slower and are not nearly as harmful to the body.

The number-one concept for good nutrition is this:

Put REAL foods into your body.

The sad truth is that most people put synthetic foods into their body and expect them to function like real foods, which they don't. A "synthetic food" is one that is highly processed and has various additives and fillers. If you are reading a food label and you cannot pronounce any word among the ingredients, put that item back on the shelf and leave it there! Don't take it home. Don't consume it.

Real foods, for the most part, are whole foods—a whole piece of fruit, preferably organically grown unless it is a piece of fruit with an impermeable "packaging" such as a banana or orange or grapefruit. As an example, choose to eat a whole apple rather than the applesauce or juice that is at the average grocery store. (The applesauce likely has ingredients that are intended to extend the shelf life of the product—not good for you ... and the juice is likely more water than juice, with way too much sugar per ounce, also not good for you. The whole apple will also give you far more fiber and a greater feeling of being "full" and satisfied than the small container of applesauce or glass of apple juice.) Whole foods include whole vegetables, of course, as well as nuts and meats from the butcher counter at the store, trimmed of excess fat.

Real foods SATISFY your body, and over time, your MIND will also find them more satisfying. At the beginning, your mind is going to resist whole foods if you aren't already eating plenty of them. You'll likely find them more bland than the fat-oozing and sugar-laced products otherwise known as "packaged" foods.

Real foods need to be eaten whenever possible in their raw state, or slightly steamed. Grilling is usually acceptable.

You can add bits of fresh herbs for flavoring, and I encourage you to experiment with herbs for "taste" variety. But don't add butter, salt, or other forms of fat to the food. And never fry the food (either deep-fat-fry or sauté in fat).

Don't just talk the talk about *wanting* to get healthier. Begin to walk the walk, and the walk begins in the grocery store and ends when you sit down to a nutritious meal, complete with a conversation with a person you love!

7. Drink sufficient water.

Divide your body weight by 2 and drink at least that many ounces of water daily. For example, if you weigh 180 pounds, you should be drinking 90 ounces of water a day. Yes, that's 11-plus small glasses. It may sound like a lot, but if you fill up a half-gallon (32-ounce) drinking glass and sip from it often during the morning, and have another full glass in the afternoon, and then another glass going to and from work and after you get home in the evening … you'll make this goal and then some!

Water is necessary for "flushing your system." In other words, it gets rid of the impurities in your body, from the cellular level on, and some of those impurities are excess fat and toxins.

Some people think that if they drink more water, they will become "bloated" or retain more water weight. The exact opposite is true. Water is actually a prime diuretic—it helps the body get *rid* of water. Essentially, adequate water intake sends a signal to the body that it does not need to hoard water, and therefore, it doesn't.

8. Get enough sleep.

The average human body needs 7–8 hours of sleep a night. Some people need a little more. Very few people can function at their best with an average of less.

I have encountered people who think sleep is a waste of time and they pride themselves on needing only a few hours of sleep a night. The truth is, they likely are doing themselves great harm—perhaps not immediately but eventually. It is during sleep that the body regenerates itself—it sloughs off toxins and replaces worn-out cells at night; it renews the immune system; and it rebalances hormones during *sleep!*

A warm bath or shower, soothing music, and reading a book of inspirational value prior to sleep may help a person get to sleep faster. Exercise during the day (no later than 2 hours before bedtime) and good nutrition all day can help a person *stay* asleep. The body does best with a dose of protein between six and eight o'clock in the evening—perhaps four ounces of non-fat cottage cheese or yogurt. This helps maintain blood sugar levels through the night, which helps a person avoid those wide-awake times that often seem to occur about four o'clock in the morning.

Notes about the EMOTIONAL Dimension of Phase 1

1. Know what "stresses you out."

Take time to reflect on your life. Consider the things that seem to result in the most stress *regularly*. One of the greatest sources of stress for many people is financial debt. The Bible has it right! ("The borrower is servant to the lender." Proverbs 22:7)

For other people, periodic outbursts of deep anger leave them feeling stressed—along with the people who witness their outbursts. For many others, an abiding frustration occurs when other people around them do not do what they promised or complete projects with high quality. Again, that frustration can be interpreted as stress!

There is yet another aspect of stress that impacts many people ... they just haven't put a label to it. The appropriate term is hyper-vigilance.

You may never have heard the term before, but hyper-vigilance is a way of saying, "Too much stimulation." It is a way of life for many people!

Certainly we all face the challenge of living with an "alert mind" open to new possibilities and opportunities, and also an "aware mind" that is quick to recognize danger or potential acts of terror. It is good for most people to be "on their toes" when it comes to work-related issues.

When, however, do alertness and awareness shift over into a genuine STRESSFUL state of hyper-vigilance?

Let's consider what happens to a person physically in times of more extreme stimulation. The response is called "sympathetic nervous system arousal," or SNS. Some people refer to this as "flight or fight" response. It can be a key to survival, but in most people in today's world, the response is just shy of what is necessary to stay alive.

The piece of lint on the floor is NOT a poisonous spider ... the shadow cast on the wall is not that of a person lurking outside the house ... the car backfire down the street is not a gunshot ... and so forth. The body, however, often does not KNOW the true nature of a stimulus and therefore, REACTS before it can make a logical and reasonable RESPONSE. The result, in SNS terms, is a release of a substance called cortisol into the system. (This is related to the adrenal gland, the source of "adrenaline," which gives a person more strength to flee or fight.) Cortisol, in turn, stimulates the production of glucose, which must be managed by an increased amount of the hormone insulin.

Those who live in a state of WORRY are especially prone to anxiety and fear. They are thus especially prone to living in a nearly constant state of low levels of cortisol being dumped into their bloodstream, including the consequences of more glucose and more insulin.

Cortisol, in and of itself, is not a culprit. It is a hormone produced as a by-product of cholesterol production. It is one of the primary stress hormones secreted from the adrenal glands and it is necessary to maintain normal internal balance and function during times of great and negative stress, including the positive stresses related to exercise and hard but satisfying physical WORK. (Positive stress can also be taxing on our system—something many people overlook). Without cortisol, the body would be unable to respond to stress. It regulates important aspects of heart rate, blood pressure, digestion, and blood sugar balance—and also our wake-sleep cycle.

If a person lives in hyper-vigilance (worry, fretting, anxiety, fear, extreme "concern") stress is nearly constant. Which means cortisol production is almost constant and eventually the adrenal glands can become exhausted. Along the way, a stressed system leads to insulin resistance, which contributes to weight gain. In addition to obesity, those with insulin resistance often experience memory loss or memory impairment, a decrease in lean body mass (loss of muscle), a decrease in bone density, an increase in anxiety, increase in depression, mood swings, decreased sexual drive or desire for intimacy, and decrease in the body's immune response and a corresponding increase in susceptibility to infection. In addition, insulin resistance has been linked to elevation in blood pressure and an alteration in hypothalamic-pituitary gland functioning, which can result in negative changes in menstruation, menopausal, and andropausal (male menopause) symptoms.

All of which leads us to conclude that insulin resistance is a state to be avoided, and this will require our dealing with anxiety and the issue of hyper-vigilance. In extreme cases, insulin resistance can lead to a body's inability to use fat as fuel, which makes weight loss almost impossible. A person's general metabolism gets totally out of whack, and there can be a dangerous increase in protein breakdown and nitrogen excretion, both of which signal a metabolizing of muscle as fuel rather than fat. The result is immune dysfunction, loss of muscle tissue, skeletal bone loss, and thinning of the skin. Low blood pressure, blood sugar imbalances, metabolic syndrome, diabetes, obesity, and even death can result.

Avoid falling in the trap! There are a number of things a person can do to avoid falling into the downward spiral of a hyper-vigilant lifestyle:

First Steps First — Phase 1

1. Maintain and foster friendships across a variety of groups.

2. Develop hobbies.

3. Take a vacation with one's family (try for an average of at least 2–3 days every 1–2 months).

4. Practice quiet introspective time for at least ten minutes a day.

5. Come to the firm conviction that you cannot change the world, or even your community. Keep things in perspective and seek to do YOUR PART.

6. Be willing to seek and receive wise counsel from a minister, licensed professional counselor, or older colleagues who have plenty of experience and compassion.

7. Be honest with yourself regarding your own tendency to be hyper-vigilant—to internalize stress in the form of anxiety, worry, fear, or in some cases, "over-caring," which is taking on too much responsibility for the lives of others.

8. Relearn the skill of relaxing—of taking a TOTAL break from the news, computers, and cell phones ... or refusing to take work home from the office ... and from being overly preoccupied with issues whose outcomes are beyond your ability to influence.

9. Make a concerted effort NOT to let worry dominate your life. Find good reasons for HOPE.

10. Refuse to give in to ever-present frustration or anger, and do not let fears take control over your life. Activate your faith!

Release the Tension. One of the best ways to release negative tension is to go for a simple walk. The chemicals produced in the brain will help metabolize the chemicals that were produced to create the "fight or flight" mentality. There is a calming of the emotions, a decrease in the intensity of brain function, and overall, a return to a state of greater inner peace and "sanity."

Nobody can immunize himself from all uncertainty and unpredictability. We can decide, however, that we are not going to live in constant fear, anxiety, or worry about the uncertain or unpredictable nature of life. We can choose to respond to moments of worry or fear in a positive way. We can *choose* to be sane.

2. Monitoring your self-talk.

What do you say to yourself, about yourself—perhaps when nobody else is around? Do you call yourself a dummy ... stupid ... klutzy ... weak ... a failure? STOP IT. You wouldn't want others to say these things about you—how dare you say them about yourself!

Even those who don't self-ridicule sometimes fall into traps of negative self-talk. One area of poor self-talk is self-entitlement—this generally is expressed as "I deserve this" ... "I *need* this and am not getting it" ... "I can't help what I WANT."

We think others owe us an easy time, and that we have a

"right" to the blessings we have been given. That generally is *not* true.

A Key to Motivation. If you think you are entitled to certain things, you likely are going to be less inclined to work for them, and to enter a blame game with others close to you. Neither is productive in the long run. These tendencies only lead to laziness and resentment from other people.

On the other hand, you *can* use self-talk in very positive ways to motivate yourself.

- Give yourself compliments. ("Hey, self, you did a good job!)

- Give yourself a pep talk. (You CAN do this. Get up and try!)

- Aim for greater excellence. (Go for the gold, baby! Don't settle for the bronze.)

- There are four motivational statements I routinely encourage my clients to make on a daily basis. Try voicing these statements aloud to your own self!

- I am unique and special ... *always.*

- I was not designed by God for defeat or failure.

- I was not created to go through life discouraged or depressed.

- I *can* achieve what I *believe* to be God's best for me.

The greatest motivator—and the most effective and trust-worthy motivator—is going to be … YOURSELF. Say what you know to be true according to God's Word and God's design for human beings. Speak the truth to yourself with deep conviction, and then take courage and ACT on what you say. Be driven from the inside.

3. Evaluate your obligations.

Countless people take on obligation after obligation without re-alizing the stress they are putting on their own lives or on their close relationships. Take a few minutes in silence—with your personal journal close at hand—to list all of the responsibilities and commitments you have. Walking the dog is not too trivial to list. Taking care of an elderly parent is a major commitment and responsibility, even if you like to think of it as an act of love or "not a problem." An obligation does not need to be problem-atic—many of our commitments are things we enjoy.

An obligation is anything others routinely expect you to do, or that you expect yourself to do.

Once you have this list made, look for areas where:

- You might delegate responsibility to someone else.

- You might negotiate a shared responsibility with someone else.

- You might be able to step away (at least temporarily) from the responsibility.

- You might be better off without the commitment. Some

tenure on committees, and some club memberships, are worthy to be "retired."

4. Let go of the weight of unforgiveness.

One of the greatest emotional weights a person can carry is unforgiveness. It preoccupies the mind and limits the emotions.

You likely *know* the name of a person or group that you have come to resent, feel deep prejudice against, or even hate. You likely can identify the bitterness, resentment, and feelings of abiding anger and frustration inside you when their name is brought into conversation. You may have a "clenching" in your spirit, and sometimes even an involuntary clenching of your fists.

Let it go! That's what forgiveness really means. It means opening the cage of your heart where you are imprisoning that person, and releasing the person—not to the general cosmos, but into the hands of God. Say aloud, "I give this problem person to You, God. Do what you want to do with them, and in them."

And then forgive yourself and move on.

Quickly Ask for Forgiveness. At times you may need to go to a person you have hurt and apologize or ask for their forgiveness. Be quick to do this. It is a strong person, not a weak one, who says, "I'm sorry."

5. Reset yourself to endure.

As implied above, feelings of entitlement leave many people feeling that all results should be quickly attained and that life should be easy. Those who feel this way are often in danger of losing all incentive to work—not just because work or the expenditure of effort is necessary to attain any significant level of achievement, refinement, or craftsmanship, but for the sheer JOY of working. There's a great deal to be said for setting a goal, and then disciplining one's self to steadily work toward that goal day in and day out, with consistency and a highly positive attitude.

Most of the things we truly value do not happen instantly. Most of the solutions we eventually experience in our lives are not "quick fix" in nature.

A problem may be solved on a sitcom in thirty minutes, a murder mystery resolved in sixty minutes. But in the real world, many problems take a lifetime to solve and true mysteries often take generations!

No really stellar relationship pops into being instantly and is maintained without effort. That's true in marriage, parenting, and also in every other form of spiritual or business relationship. Consistency over time—and consistently doing the right things, and pursuing the right goals—is a must.

A number of years ago, I saw a sign in a restaurant: "We are not a fast-food joint. We are a slow-food establishment. It takes us many hours to prepare our meats and the side dishes that go with them. We ask you to be patient for a few minutes so we can prepare them for delivery to your table with the quality of service they deserve." I loved eating there!

Show me a place that specializes in "microwave" food and I'll show you a place that likely sells lots of antacids and digestive aids just an aisle away.

All of this leads to a simple conclusion: You may need to adjust your expectations when it comes to how quickly you will be able to reach your goals.

Slow Down and Get Real. We live in a culture that seems to love speed! We not only want fast food and fast service, but we look for the thrill associated with fast cars, fast amusement-park rides, fast change, and results and remedies, and fast relationships that we expect to have lasting value.

Fast does not always satisfy!

Life is a marathon, not a sprint. The best things in life are sometimes SLOW.

Start. And keep going. And don't quit. That's the only way to get to a finish line that you will be glad to cross!

Notes about the INTELLECTUAL Dimension of Phase 1

1. Learn something!

I'm not at all saying that a person cannot "learn" from reading fiction, especially historical fiction. BUT real learning comes mostly from reading and studying nonfiction. Nonfiction sources can include biographies, theories (presented as programs, plans), and scientific research. It comes in the form of books, journal articles, and "briefs."

Many short courses can also qualify as learning "events" that don't take longer than reading a serious nonfiction book. If you want to "listen" to your nonfiction, feel free to do so.

The brain was designed for thinking just as
the body was designed for movement.

Refuse to be discouraged. Continual learning is one of the best ways I know to stay encouraged about the world.

We each must fight the tendency NOT to be discouraged by the overwhelming amount of information available in our world today. Sample information broadly, but recognize that your greatest satisfaction is going to be the study of *something* until you get to the point of mastery.

Read history in order to LEARN from it.

Read the biographies of great men and women to be INSPIRED by their examples.

Read science to be retain your SENSE OF AWE at the beauties of God's creation and the new studies that may lead to cures of currently incurable diseases, the innovations that can make life easier for the disabled, the inventions that are on the horizon that enhance our ability to connect with others, and the new horizons that are unfolding for research and technological invention.

Read spiritual literature—I recommend the Holy Bible—to tap into real TRUTH.

Refuse to Be Gullible. As you read, ask questions. Actively engage your own rational thinking processes. Refuse to be gullible. Not everything you read is going to be truth.

Several years ago I tried a little experiment.

I put out three testimonial statements on a social media outlet. I gave a paragraph to a 41-year-old man who told how much body fat he had lost in four weeks, and about the drop in inches around his belly. I gave another paragraph to a 34-year-old female who was thrilled at her weight loss in only 6 weeks with "no dieting or exercise." She was exceedingly happy to be ready for her new bikini by the time of her summer beach trip. I then gave a paragraph to a 53-year-old male who was very glad for a weight loss plan that didn't require time for exercise or a diet plan. He told me how many people he had recruited to my wonderful new product that was called NOW & FOREVER YOUNG.

This product, I explained, was new, natural, safe, and effective. It was a dietary supplement that came from a remote village of Hawaiian people on the big island of Hawaii. I had discovered the product on my first visit there several years ago and was amazed at the physiques and health of the general population. When I asked what this people did to have such beautifully sculpted lean bodies I was told that they spent NO time in gyms, ate plenty of fried and fatty foods, and for the most part, had a relatively sedentary lifestyle. There was only ONE thing they had in common. They all ate pineapple seeds. These were not ordinary pineapple seeds—they were only found in the pineapples found in a grove near their village.

I discovered the location of this grove and began to eat these seeds myself. I couldn't believe the positive results I experienced!

I then let the readers of this social network site know I had secured exclusive rights to distribute the extract from these seeds in water-soluble capsules, approved by physicians, and that study after study had confirmed the tremendous weight-loss benefits of this product. Supplies were limited so I was only able to let my friends have access to the product. A six-month supply could be had for $89.93. And then I added, "God bless you in your pursuit of health."

I only left this fairly short article on the site for 72 hours, and I assure you every word of the article was "legal." You may be surprised, but the FDA will allow most messages about health-related products as long as they do not claim that a product "treats, cures, or prevents disease or illness."

I was totally blown away by the response I received from only 72 hours of no-promotion information on one small site. I received more than $3,000 in orders in 48 hours.

Yes … it was a scam. I didn't take any of the money offered to me for the product and I didn't ship any extract from pineapple seeds. The entire experiment was something I did to see just how gullible the population can be. I got my answer. The world clamors for a quick-fix, takes-no-effort protocol for losing weight and getting a lean body.

I didn't do this to make anyone feel foolish. It was designed to educate and inform. I sent a message loud and clear to all who responded:

- If something sounds too good to be true in the area of exercise and nutrition, it is.

- If something says "all natural," that doesn't mean it is safe. Rattlesnake venom is all natural.

- If it requires urgent response—act now or forever lose your chance at a limited supply—run away from the "opportunity."

- If the information says it has a physician's blessing, write and ask for the physician's credentials.

- If the article has testimonials, realize that anyone can write a testimonial—it doesn't mean it is *their* actual experience.

- Eating fattening food and living a sedentary life will increase a person's chances of illness and a great quality of life over time. You can't get lean and healthy without a little restraint and effort.

- Having a healthy body and mind ALWAYS requires effort, dedication, and commitment. Nothing of real value comes easy.

A sad commentary on those who wrote back—they were dismayed that there was no pineapple-seed product and they didn't at all appreciate my "lecture" about health. In other words, they WANTED the lie to be true ... and they wanted the truth of what I had to say to be a lie.

That's a dangerous perspective to adopt!

2. Mini vacations are good to take.

Close the door, put your head down on your desk or lean back in your sofa, and imagine a place of great beauty, serenity, and pleasurable sights, sounds, and aromas. Spend five minutes there.

The place you imagine may be somewhere you have been … or someplace you'd like to visit. It can be a beach, mountain, or populated setting.

See the place in your mind as vividly as possible—imagine all the colors, textures, and various sensual stimuli that you can!

Enjoy the experience. And then get back to work!

You'll find that a mini vacation is motivating, and that it often breaks the monotony of a boring task to the point that you *can* return to the task and do it faster, more efficiently, and with less frustration.

Fantasize only good. There's no joy, however, in going to a "place" that is going to create in you a desire for sin or that causes you any sort of pain.

Be careful in your choice of imaginary companions in your mini-vacation place. This is not intended to be an X-rated, adulterous, or pornographic venture. Keep it pure. Keep it lovely. Keep it unsullied.

3. Single task.

For the past several decades, "multi-tasking" has been a popular idea. Finding ways of doing two things at the same time speaks to our desire for "doing more in less time" and being supremely efficient. The problem: research is showing that it is not all that efficient and that people often don't accomplish nearly as much as they think they are accomplishing.

The better approach is to learn to focus on *one task* and get it finished, and then move on to the next task. Don't let yourself be interrupted. Stay steady in your effort. You don't need to hurry—you just need to be diligent.

Try it and see how much MORE you might get done in an hour … or a day.

Notes about the SPIRITUAL Dimension of Phase 1

1. The joy of silence.

Are you comfortable being alone and silent?

Are you comfortable being with another person and remaining silent?

Silence is important. It is the "space" in which we gain perspective, and are able to most adequately "shift gears" from one task to another or from one idea to another. It is a place that often gives rise to great creativity and innovation. Seek to cultivate silence in your life.

The recommendation in the Wellness Plan is for 10 minutes of silence in a day. For some people, that's a real stretch. If 10 minutes sounds like a long time, start with just ONE minute. But if you will take the challenge of remaining absolutely silent during a full minute, you may have a new appreciation for just how long a minute can be!

Eliminate all the noise you can control. (You cannot do anything about natural noise from wind, rain, and so forth.) Turn off your cell phone, your computer, all music, television, and "people sounds." This may mean shutting a door or two. Try to get away from any neighborhood sounds such as leaf blowers or traffic noise.

I know a person who goes to the new "safe room" they had installed in their garage. He closes the door and just "sits" there for a minute or two ... or sometimes for five to ten minutes. He calls it his "decompression capsule," and in many ways, a time in total silence does serve as a decompression experience.

Take Every Thought Captive. In silence, you face a very real challenge of taking every thought "captive." What you choose to think about in silence is important—and is the real *reason* for silence as part of a wellness perspective.

This is not just a matter of turning off the television set or CD player. Those things are only a BEGINNING. (Most newcomers to "quiet time" aren't disciplined enough to shut out all noise without actually shutting off the noise makers!)

Quiet time is rooted in the idea of turning off all external stimuli, including thoughts related to the mundane chores and responsibilities of life. This is a time NOT to think about your list of things to do, your undone chores, or your grocery list. It is a time for reflecting on those things that you think are truly important in life and that are the "best ideas" worth thinking.

One of the writers of the New Testament said that a person is wise to think about things that are:

- True — not fiction or fantasy, and not speculation or idle gossip, but genuine reality that has an eternal quality to it

- Noble — the best and highest of ideals about how to live personally, how to relate to God, and how to relate to other people

- Just — principles and practices that are equitable and appropriate for all people at all times in all cultures

- Pure — moral according to God's commandments

- Lovely — beautiful, attractive in their innocence

- Good report — all things considered praiseworthy and virtuous (See Philippians 4:8.)

A person once said to me, "I'm not sure I can define what these thoughts might be … but I think it would probably be good for me to try to define those words and come up with as many examples as I can!" I couldn't agree more.

So much of what we think about in any given day seems to be rooted in the trivial. It is a wonderful "escape" from the mundane moments of life to think about things that truly have the potential for eternal reward or the productive of earthly blessings.

Quiet-time thinking is often a matter of an increased focus on gratitude—listing or thinking about what causes you to feel truly *thankful* and blessed. It is also a matter of placing increased importance on praise—what you acknowledge as the lasting and ultimate qualities of God, not just for now but for all eternity, as well as what you consider to be the lasting legacy of people you most admire and desire to emulate (both living and dead).

Yoga? Meditation? Prayer?

The various methodologies for establishing "quiet" in a person's life are varied. Yoga is generally a series of positions, usually accompanied by concepts. (Original yoga is a set of positions for Buddhist prayer, but non-Buddhist variations have been created.)

Meditation is generally a means of "focus" that includes breathing techniques to quiet the body and the mind simultaneously.

Prayer is a matter of communing with God and includes adoration, thanksgiving, praise, confession of sin, and making petitions—often with a focus on just one or two of these practices at any given time.

I personally choose prayer as my method for enjoying a quiet time because it is in keeping with my spiritual beliefs, and it is something I have been comfortable doing for decades. Prayer for me is ultimately a simple matter of talking to God, and of spending time *listening* for God to reply. Ideally, I find that I am benefitted most by spending at LEAST as much time listening as I do talking.

Does God talk to people? Most assuredly. But a person has to be listening to hear Him! God doesn't usually talk in an audible voice, at least not to *most* people, but He does speak through impressions, ideas, and feelings that are felt deep within a person's spirit. It takes some time to quiet one's mind and heart in order to "hear" those messages ... but that's the very purpose of a quiet time!

Any form of "quieting the mind" can have benefit for a person. But be aware that this isn't just a matter of "thinking." Too often "thinking" becomes a time for worrying, of trying to solve problems in relationships, or of trying to figure out solutions for needs. Quiet-time thoughts and feelings are more like "thinking and feeling without an agenda."

2. Deep breathing cleanses toxins.

I have put deep breathing in the spiritual dimension of Phase 1 because it has a two-fold result. While it is a major way of cleansing the lungs, and thus, the bloodstream, of toxins, it is also a way of cleansing one's spiritual perspective if you do it this way:

• As you *INHALE*, envision yourself taking in all of God's goodness and love.

• As you *EXHALE,* envision yourself releasing all of the negative   emotions you may be harboring.

This makes deep breathing a form of prayer!

Use Your Diaphragm. The diaphragm is a curved muscular membrane that separates your abdomen from the area around your lungs. Think of it as a superb "breathing muscle."

Most people begin and end their breathing by using shoulder muscles—breathing is an "up and down" event for them. Diaphragmatic breathing (deep breathing) is an "in and out" event. This type of breathing forces a response from the Parasympathetic Nervous System. The parasympathetic nervous system produces what many call the "relaxation" response that promotes a *decrease* in blood pressure, heart rate, respiration, adrenaline production, muscle tension, and perspiration.

Here's how this type of breathing is done:

1. Lie flat on your back with your hands resting on your abdomen (near your naval).

2. As you inhale, force your abdomen to push upward (as if opening your lungs to take in all the oxygen it can hold).

3. As you exhale, move your abdomen back downward (as if pushing out all the air that has been inhaled).

4. When you begin to get a rhythm with this, put a little resistance (with your hands) against your abdomen as you push it up and then back down during your breathing. Do this for at least one minute.

Breathe in as deeply as you can.

Exhale as much of the air in your lungs as you can.

Most people can do about six DEEP breathing cycles (in and out) in a minute. And that's enough to arouse the parasympathetic nervous system into action. In fact, a beginner should probably not try to do more than six deep breaths in a cycle.

Doing this two to three times a day, several hours apart, can make a tremendous difference in your efforts to control stress levels!

3. Reading for spiritual enrichment.

I personally do not know of a greater written source of spiritual enrichment than the Bible. It contains TRUTH, not just good ideas. The reading of it builds up faith, confidence in God's love, and a desire to love others as nothing else I have ever encountered. The Bible challenges a person to grow spiritually, and presents a very clear understanding about what *God* considers to be right and wrong.

If you are new to Bible reading, I recommend that you start with the Gospels, the first four "books" in the New Testament. Also read the Psalms and the Proverbs. Branch out into the first couple books of the Old Testament and relive the great "Bible stories" you may have heard as a child. Don't get discouraged if you don't understand everything you read—just keep reading. You may find it helpful to find a version of the Bible that is in modern-day language (as opposed to the old King James language of "thee" and "thou"). Spend 10 minutes a day in the Bible and you will be amazed at all you will learn over the course of a month.

There are many other deeply spiritual books written by great men and women through the ages. You may want to ask a clerk in a Bible bookstore to direct you to truly "classic" writings that can help a person grow spiritually. You'll likely be amazed at all that is available.

4. Share your faith with others.

Make friends with people who believe what you believe. You will find that these are your *greatest* friends if you encounter a personal or family crisis. Friends with a depth of spirituality are people you generally can trust to be a positive influence on your children. They are often friends to whom you can turn for advice or wise counsel. If you desire to have a mentor or accountability partner in your life, choose a person who shares your value system and believes what you believe.

My Sharing of Faith with You. As author and reader, we are in the process of developing something of a "relationship." And since that relationship has a spiritual dimension, I believe it only right for you as a reader to have an opportunity to know a little more about me if you are going to be evaluating any spiritual "coaching" I may offer to you. If I could summarize my spiritual journey in one word it would be TRUST. From my earliest days, I knew that the only person I truly could TRUST in life was God. And I discovered early on that God was utterly trustworthy. He was always true to His Word and always available with His help.

I was adopted as a baby and did not have any awareness or relationship with my "birth mother" until well into my adult years. I'm very grateful to the couple who adopted me as their only child—they were a true mom and dad in every way. But like many adopted children, I always felt a little "outside" the deep intimacy of relationships—something was missing that I could never quite understand or overcome. As a boy, I was weaker and smaller than many of the "cool" kids in my grade, and I also had somewhat large ears that always seemed to be the brunt of peer jokes. I endured the ridicule I received and did my best to ignore it, but I had a big reservoir or inner pain most of my growing-up years.

On the positive side, I was always considered to be a "nice guy." That didn't necessarily translate into popularity, or dates with cute girls, but it did give me fewer problems related to teasing when I entered my teen years. I'm grateful to the parents who taught me to be kind, polite, and show respect to others.

Also as a big plus, I was athletically gifted and my sport of choice was baseball. I did an "acceptable" job in the academic area of life, but I put my major effort and passion into being the best baseball player I could be in order to get a scholarship to college. That happened. And I gave the same effort to baseball in college with the hope of a professional career. I did manage to earn a business degree in the process, and I'm very grateful that baseball gave me that "added benefit" for my life and career in the years that followed college.

I was offered a job playing professional baseball in the South Australia Baseball League. I was recruited as a catcher, and I was an active player in many games. I had a great deal of spare time during any given day and I decided to spend that time in a local gym, and to try lifting weights—something that I had never pursued before. That experience drastically changed my life.

When I returned to the United States, I joined the law enforcement ranks as a police officer. A good physique was an asset in that career, and I continued the weight lifting. I also discovered that I was suddenly more attractive to the opposite sex as a man with strong muscles! Because of my inexperience in the dating world, I made many mistakes. Even though I found myself married and divorced twice by the time I was in my thirties, I was and still am determined to be the best father possible to my three wonderful children. And I am happy to report that I finally got it "right" in the marriage department—my wife Michele is a blessing beyond anything I can describe.

I have had many other setbacks in my life and have experienced the destructive power of untrue words. I learned the truth of the old saying, "Trying to undo a rumor is like trying to unring a bell." Further, I continue to learn many lessons about maintaining one's integrity and living a quiet, patient, consistent life during that time.

One of the most shocking heartbreaks of my life occurred when my mother, who had suffered from depression for many years, took her own life. My heart still breaks when I recall that event. My father, who is still alive, was also deeply affected and still suffers.

I do not share these experiences with you to try to gain sympathy, but rather, when I tell you that I learned to TRUST God you will know that my faith was not my last resort during difficult times but my FIRST resort. I am grateful that I was raised in a home where church attendance was the norm. I am grateful that I made a decision to trust God early in my life. I am grateful that I can turn to God every day and trust Him to help me develop the WELLNESS that He desires for me—first and foremost, spiritual wellness, but also an overall growth toward the "wholeness" that is God's best design for every person.

Over the years, I learned that my trust of God translated into an ability to receive God's forgiveness, to forgive other people, and to forgive myself. It also translated into an ability to love others without expecting their love in return. I wouldn't want to live any other way—trusting God, living in a *state* of forgiveness, and living with love in my heart is the best possible approach to life I can imagine. And if I had to summarize Spiritual Wellness in three statements it would be these:

- Trust God.

- Forgive freely, and receive forgiveness. When you know that you are forgiven by God, forgive yourself and move forward with courage.

- Choose to love others—to give to them generously and to pray for them—without requiring anything in return.

5

NUGGETS OF
INFORMATION AND
INSPIRATION

(AS YOU MOVE FROM PHASE 1 TO PHASE 2)

NOW IS THE TIME for consolidation and balance!

Several essays are included in the pages that follow. They are intended to inform you about key areas of wellness that apply to most people. They are also intended to inspire you and motivate you to remain committed to the changes that are reflected in your personal goals.

As you read through, note, and reflect on this information, expect to be challenged. And then do these three things:

1. Reflect on what you have written in your journal. Be grateful for your progress and find a healthful way to

reward yourself for the GOOD things you are implementing in your life.

2. Review your goals and "reset" them if need be. Some behaviors may have been more difficult to turn into regular habits. You may want to set some sub-goals.

3. Renew your commitment to wellness! Remain intentional, focused, and disciplined. You CAN do this!

Nuggets

1. Getting Fit Is a Long-Term Process

I have been active in the fitness industry and in bodybuilding for decades. I once traveled and spoke with a group of body-builders—we called ourselves The Power Team. Let it suffice to say that I have well-developed muscles!

This obvious physical trait has led a number of people to ask me through the years, "Do you take steroids?" I used to be offended at that question. The question seemed to imply to me that I was either doing something illegal (which the use of steroids can be), or that I was "cheating" in some way. The people who asked this question rarely knew that I worked for many years in law enforcement, and I was a "good cop" who did NOT engage in illegal activities. I sought to keep the letter of the law and did not ignore the spirit of the law. There are no shortcuts in the concept of hard work.

I got over being offended in this area. Now I just answer the question as politely as I can: "No, I don't take steroids. I take two hours at the gym several days a week, and have done that for more than twenty-five years."

I am surprised at times to see that people are disappointed at my answer. They seem to WANT to believe that a body's muscles can be "built up" by taking drugs—it's a quick fix, perhaps, that they might try someday?

During most weeks, I work out with weights for six hours a week and do six hours of aerobics training. That's twelve hours a week. I've done this for twenty-five years. There's a word for this kind of effort: WORK. But before you think I've gone way overboard, let me assure you that I live a very balanced life. I travel a great deal, get 7–8 hours of sleep a night, spend time in quality relationships, and do my "day job" with consistent dedication, commitment, and high output. I spend time learning and time in prayer every day. Another way of looking at the exercise commitment: Of the 168 hours in any given week (7 days x 24 hours), I *only* spend 12 hours a week in focused, well-planned exercise. That's only seven percent of my time. In comparison, I spend almost thirty percent of my time in deep and restful sleep and about forty percent of my time in career-related work!

Because I work in the area of wellness education and counseling, I also see my time in the gym as directly related to my work. I do not feel at all comfortable telling any person *what* to do unless I know from personal experience that my advice works. I am determined to be the best role model I know how to be when it comes to wellness.

At the same time, let me quickly say that I am telling you this at the outset of discussing the emotional, intellectual, and spiritual aspects of wellness because I am thoroughly convinced that these three dimensions of wellness are just as important, if not more so, than the physical aspects of wellness associated with nutrition and exercise. Furthermore, I firmly believe that the physical aspects of wellness *contribute* to a person's ability to maximize their pursuit of the emotional, intellectual, and spiritual dimensions of life.

Things of Value Take Time. Not long ago I heard about a man in his late fifties who was honored by the local blood bank as one of their highest donors over a three-decade period. He had given many gallons of blood in his life. You can't do that in a day, week, month, or year.

I also met a woman not long ago who does major needlework projects for churches. Each canvas she works takes hundreds of hours to design and complete. The result is stunningly beautiful. But that kind of craftsmanship and beauty doesn't happen in a day, week, month, or year.

I know of a man who has created a phenomenal Japanese garden on the two acres of his backyard high in the mountains above the Palm Springs desert. It took him twenty-five years to train the plants in the authentic manner of Japanese horticulture. The result is intricate and complicated and truly awe-inspiring. It is not the work that can be done in a day, a week, a month, or a year.

Any body of professional work and contribution to society takes time.

The development of a person's spiritual life takes a LIFETIME.

Do Things You Can ENJOY for a Lifetime. We rarely try to short-circuit a process if we truly enjoy that process!

Have I enjoyed every hour in the gym? No. But I've enjoyed most of them, and I nearly always leave the gym after a work-out feeling good about the time spent there and the work done there.

Does my friend the needlework designer enjoy stitching? She tells me it would be her hobby if it wasn't her work. And the same for the man growing a true Japanese garden—he truly enjoys the planning, pruning, and design associated with his work.

Choose to enjoy what you do. And don't hurry the results.

Take time to delight in the EFFORT and the journey.

As a friend of mine once said, "If you travel at night so you can go 80 miles an hour toward your destination, you may get there by dawn, but you'll fail to see the beauty of the area through which you traveled."

2. Give Up Your Excuses

The best thing you can do with excuses is "give them up!" As a part of monitoring your self-talk, pay special attention to your voicing of excuses.

Through the years I've discovered that excuses are almost as numerous as the people who rely on them:

- I don't have time.

- I don't see any beneficial purpose in doing this.

- I know I'll fail so why begin?

- I don't think this is important for ME.

- I will start tomorrow (or next week or next month …).

Whatever excuse you are using … it really isn't a good justification for *choosing* to live short of your wellness potential!

The longer you make excuses instead of making positive changes, the longer you will fall short of your potential for more energy and strength. There's no other conclusion that can be rationally drawn.

The more you shunt responsibility for your wellness to someone else, the more you are sending a signal to others around you that you don't *care* if you become a health-care burden on them.

3. Seek to Become Proactive about Nutrition

In getting nutritionally savvy, you need to:

- Educate yourself about foods—including vitamins, minerals, and supplements.

- Consult a nutritionist about what you need to eat and how much of it (the nutritionist might be a "virtual" one found on a DVD series, or in a book … it is often a good shortcut to talk with someone who is a licensed nutritionist—just one appointment can put you on the right track).

- Create a weight-loss plan—with both short-term and

long-term goals that are both realistic for you and motivating to you.

Make Decisions about Your Eating and Act on Them. As you start out in revamping the way you eat, make two key decisions and then stick to them:

- Commit to eating one meal a day that is "totally healthy."

- Commit to eating at scheduled times in a day—not at random or after you are already ravenous.

- Those two choices cost NOTHING to make, and they can make a huge difference.

- The next two decisions are a little more difficult—as in, they take a little more time and a planning:

- Have healthy foods available for snacking. Whether you are in your office or car, it helps to have a couple of healthy meal replacement bars, trail mix, and fruit handy.

- Have plenty of water nearby at all times. Keep a bottle of water in a desk drawer or in your car at all times. And then, drink it! Keep your body hydrated all day—just four ounces every hour will mean sufficient water during a day. This not only helps stave off hunger, but it helps with digestion and elimination.

If healthy food and water are available and visible, you will eat and drink what is good for you! If it isn't available and visible, you'll turn to other foods that are likely going to send you on a sugar roller-coaster or leave you feeling unsatisfied and craving more.

4. Discover WHO Motivates You

Motivation isn't always a matter of WHAT motivates you. It can be a matter of WHOM.

I have three wonderful children whom I love dearly. I want each one of them to excel as a human being and experience true joy during their years on this earth. When they make great choices, I try to reaffirm in them what I believe about them and for them.

My children are part of what motivates ME to be the best person I can be. I want to be a good role model for them, but also earn the right to be an "authority" on success. That way, when I offer my praise or affirmation, it has greater weight!

Part of my ability to give credible praise and affirmation to others lies in my ability to give credible praise and affirmation to myself.

I know when I do well. Don't you know that about *yourself*?

I know when I mess up a little, or even fail miserably. You likely know that about yourself as well.

I know that when I do well, it is acceptable for me to compliment my own self and to give thanks to God for giving me the ability and opportunity to do well. I don't take all the credit for any accomplishment—if God didn't give me the strength, energy, the next beat of my heart and the next breath of my lungs, I couldn't do *anything*. I know that and I freely acknowledge it.

It is only one more step to thanking God for every moment of "good results" that I experience. And at the same time, request His help in producing more good results!

I know that when I fail, it is not God who set me up for failure. I'm pretty good at failing all on my own. I have full confidence, however, that God stands ready to pick me up, answer all of my questions about why I failed and what I might do to avoid failing in the future, and to assist me step by step as I walk in the direction He leads me.

Along the way, my setting of goals is in this context of my DESIRE to be the best person I can be—not only for the sake of my children and others who watch my life, not only for my own sense of self-value, but also as part of my giving honor to my Creator.

The setting of goals is something that I do very intentionally, but it is not an activity that is void of consultation. The keys for me are these:

- I ask God what HE desires for me to achieve and do.

- I ask God to show me WHO He has put into my life for me to influence or help.

And then …

- I ask God to help me achieve the most and influence mightily!

5. The Management of Treasure and Success

Goals are vital to the maximum management of:

- **Treasure**. I prefer this word to money. Treasure includes all things a person considers highly valuable—including material items (precious metal, gems, stocks and bonds, property and real estate investments)—relationships, work accomplishments that are influential and beneficial to society, and ministry projects to which the person contributes regularly or substantially. Treasure can be thought of in terms of a goal's CONTENT. It is the VALUE of a goal—the long-range or eternal purpose of having a goal.

- **Success**. Success is the accomplishment of an aim or purpose, including the attainment of popularity or profit. Success is the STRATEGY for attaining that goal. It is the how-to that drives a person to pursue a goal.

I recently spoke at a school and then later that same day, at another event. There was a young woman present at both functions. She saw me at the second event and in the midst of the crowd, she approached me, hugged me, looked me in the eyes, and said "thank you." She then went on to tell me about the hope and encouragement I had given her.

Is that moment one that I cherish? Yes. It is a memory that speaks to the very content of the goals I had set for those two speaking events.

It also was a moment that told me the *strategy* I had used in preparing my lectures worked.

If you ask me what to expect from goal-setting, my answer is now this: Set a goal that truly will represent treasure to you once it is achieved, and also validate the strategies or methods that you are employing in your life and in the pursuit of your goals. Have a clear understanding of both the WHAT and HOW questions related to your goals.

6. Get Serious about Your Weight

Get serious about your weight. Many people think they are just a "little heavy" when, in scientific terms, they are actually obese. An increasing number of people in our society are morbidly obese. Notice that word *morbidly*—it means "deadly." Morbidity is a term used to describe death rate, and that applies to millions of Americans—they are death waiting to happen.

I'm not intending to scare you … well, maybe a little. Obesity, of all the factors related to the most deadly diseases in our culture (heart attacks, strokes, diabetes, cancer), is the one factor that can be reversed in nearly all cases over a six-month to one-year period.

The Dangers of Overeating. I try to stay out of restaurants that offer "All You Can Eat." That's a little like saying to me, "Come and Be a Glutton Here." Gluttony is an insatiable appetite for something that can never bring fullness or satisfaction—it relates to many areas of life, not only eating and drinking.

There are very real physical detriments to overeating:

1. Your stomach can only hold so much. If you stretch it beyond its limits, your digestion process will become far less efficient.

2. During the eating process, the body and mind feel an immediate sense of gratification (or happiness). Overeating produces an even longer sense of remorse of feeling "bad" (as in bloated, lethargic, too full).

3. The stomach is made a certain size for a reason. If we take in too much for the body to process the food as energy, it turns the excess intake to fat.

4. Eating too much promotes obesity, which can contribute to heart problems, diabetes, high blood pressure, and joint pain. Portion size and overeating are two of the major causes of the obesity epidemic in our culture.

5. Overeating can become habitual, often making a person a "slave to food." Many people have no idea the number of calories they consume in a day, or even in a meal. They are usually surprised to find that they are eating at least twenty percent more than their body needs in any given meal, and over a day, many people are eating almost twice as many calories as their body needs. The excess becomes fat unless the person is on an extreme exercise program.

6. Bad eating habits can lead to food addictions—craving certain foods or categories of foods with frequent binge eating or overeating. Food addiction is harder to break than an addiction to alcohol and drugs. The best approach is not to overeat in the first place.

7. Gluttony causes many people to lose sight of the fact that having sufficient food is a *blessing*. We are very fortunate to live in a land that has plenty, rather than a land with not enough. If we lose sight of those in the world who do not have enough food, we can become callous in our hearts and less compassionate. Is there a body-spirit connection? Absolutely.

8. Food is designed primarily to fuel the body, not to give "pleasure." The key food measurement is the "calorie," which is a unit of ENERGY. This isn't to say that we cannot or should not enjoy the taste of our food. It is to say that if we are only eating for pleasure, we can quickly lose sight of the real reason for eating.

All that TASTES good or looks tasty ... isn't truly GOOD for you!

I not only encourage people to think about what they are eating, but also think about:

- How much they are eating. Be conscious and intentional about how much food you put on a plate. Some people find it very helpful to use a dessert plate or a "luncheon plate" instead of a major dinner plate, for all meals. And then, only fill that plate once and don't go back for "seconds."

It also helps some people to avoid eating in courses. Have any appetizer or salad or soup served or brought to the table at the same time as the main course. This gives a much more accurate visual picture of how much food is available.

- How they talk about food. Do you describe certain dishes as "heaven in the mouth"? Most people *desire* to go to heaven one day in the distant future; we feel certain the feasting there will be grand; but most people also believe that our body in heaven will not be a physical one that requires calories or is subject to gluttony. If you truly want heaven to be present on this earth in your life, be accurate in the way you think about and describe heaven!

At the same time, watch how you talk about overeating. There are people who brag or joke about how much they eat or about eating "too much" as if it is a badge of honor. It isn't.

Did God Make You Fat? I have overheard people say, "God made me this way [referring to their overweight body]. You just need to love me and accept me the way I am."

I love people. I do accept them. But I do not believe God *makes* people obese, sick, or lazy. Those are choices made with the *human* will.

Obesity leads to having less energy and strength, and in turn, less motivation, less "drive" to do great things in life, and less effectiveness in doing basic tasks and taking personal responsibility for one's actions. Obesity can be reversed. People can and do lose the weight necessary to restore energy and strength! They nearly always feel a renewed zest for living when they do so. They begin to dream bigger dreams, attempt to accomplish more good goals, and feel greater hope for their own future.

Sickness is not God's will—in more than eighty percent of all cases, sickness is related to poor lifestyle choices in a person's past, perhaps as long as ten or more years ago. Some sicknesses are part of a genetic pattern passed down through generations.

Most chronic illness is related to behavior, not genes. One research study concluded with very clear statistical backup that more than seventy percent of all major chronic illnesses in our nation could be eliminated or greatly reduced if we stopped smoking and using heavy-duty illegal drugs or pain medicines, stopped drinking alcohol, and embarked on more nutritional eating and exercise patterns. Sickness can often be turned into health!

Laziness is not God's will. God has given each person a free will for making most of the decisions and choices required for wellness, and for having a right relationship with Him. In addition, God's Word says that every person has been given a measure of faith—or the ability to *believe*—which includes believing for a better future and a change in circumstances. It is up to each person, therefore, to activate his or her own will and faith, and the good news is that when a person does so, God nearly always provides added spiritual power so that our will becomes true *willpower*, and our faith becomes true life-changing spiritual energy! You likely cannot motivate a lazy person to get up and get going … but if you are the lazy person in question, you *can* motivate yourself to get moving in a positive direction!

Rate of Weight Loss. Do not attempt to lose more than 8 pounds a month, or 2 pounds a week. Great results can accrue over time if you only lose one pound a month! That's 12 pounds in a year, and if you stick with it, that can easily be 50 pounds in five years. Sound like a long way away? Well, in all likelihood, you got into an obese state over a *long* time—month by month, bit by bit.

> A habit of overeating can indicate an eating disorder, or a food addiction. A food addiction is harder to break than an addiction to alcohol or drugs. And an eating disorder can be deadly if it isn't diagnosed and remedied!

7. Here's to a Healthy Heart!

Heart ailments are the number one cause of death for both men and women in the United States. A great deal can be done to reduce coronary artery disease (CAD), heart attacks that result from CAD, and other risk factors that are related to strokes (a cardiovascular "attack" that hits the brain rather than the heart).

The eight major causes of CAD are:

1. Abnormal blood cholesterol. A goal of total cholesterol should be 200 or less. A number between 200 and 239 is borderline high and a total of 240 or more is high.

2. Hypertension (high blood pressure). Normal is an average of less than 120/80, 130–139/80-89 being pre-hypertensive, and 140–159/90-99 being stage one hypertension (medical urgency). If a person has a blood pressure of 160+/100+ that is considered stage two hypertension (medical emergency).

3. Tobacco use—of all kinds.

4. Pre-diabetes. A normal fasting blood glucose level should be 70–99/dl.

5. Family history of heart disease. If a male blood relative had a history of CAD prior to age 55, or a female with a similar diagnosis prior to age 65, a person likely has a genetic link to CAD.

6. A sedentary lifestyle. A lack of moderate intensity physical activity can lead to CAD.

7. Obesity. The easiest indicator is a waist-to-hip ratio greater than 1.0 in males and .8 in females.

8. Age. Males over the age of 45 and females over the age of 55 are most prone to CAD.

Now, what can be done? A GREAT DEAL!

Let's take the eight categories above and put some helpful suggestions with them:

1. Cholesterol
   - Increase physical activity
   - Make better nutritional choices
   - Decrease body fat
   - Manage stress better
   - Control diabetes
   - Stop using tobacco products

2. Hypertension (same suggestions as cholesterol above)

3. Tobacco use
   - Stop using all tobacco products! *NOW!*

4. Prediabetes
   - Increase physical activity
   - Make better nutritional choices
   - Decrease body fat

5. Family history
   - We can't change this one, but we can face up to the truth that we must *compensate* for our family history as best we can.

6. A sedentary lifestyle
   - Increase physical activity
   - Make better nutritional choices
   - Decrease body fat
   - Manage stress better

7. Obesity
   - Increase physical activity
   - Make better nutritional choices
   - Decrease body fat
   - Manage stress better

8. Age
   - Can't change this one. But we can face the truth that the older we get, the more important it is to seek WELLNESS!

I know you saw the repeated admonitions to increase physical activity, make better nutritional choices, decrease body fat, and manage stress better.

It should also be obvious that you can have great impact on six of the eight major contributors to heart disease. Some instances of CAD are not preventable, but many are! You make the call ... I strongly urge you to be proactive in this and opt for prevention rather than hope for later recovery.

8. Tips for Dining Out

Although I am a huge advocate for cooking and eating at home, I do eat out occasionally, and I choose NOT to "cheat" when I do so.

1. I do not eat the free bread and chips that are often offered by a restaurant as a "first course." These foods promote a high insulin spike, which signals the body to store fat. Both bread and chips are very poor in nutritional value.

2. I choose a reasonable portion of lean protein, baked or grilled. I especially enjoy tilapia, salmon, chicken breast, and lean steak (beef or bison).

3. I choose a mixed green salad but make sure the dressing is kept on the side. The best dressing, if any, is a simple vinegar and oil dressing. I put the tongs of my fork in the dressing before I load that fork with greens. This cuts down sharply on the amount of dressing I use.

4. I choose grilled or steamed vegetables, with any topping or butter on the side. (I use the same technique with the butter that I use with salad dressing.)

5. I avoid white potatoes, or choose sweet potatoes (or red skin potatoes with the skin still on). White potatoes are very high on the Glycemic Index, but the other two potato types are only moderately glycemic.

6. I drink plenty of water with my meal. This helps promote a full feeling and curbs overeating.

7. I chew my food slowly and thoroughly. This helps with the digestive process. It takes the stomach twenty minutes to send a strong signal to the brain that the stomach has received sufficient food. That's a long time, especially in a restaurant. This delayed, but normal, physical response is one of the major reasons people overeat.

8. I avoid dessert (usually desserts are loaded with sugar and have a very high glycemic number).

9. I avoid all fried foods.

10. I eliminate the term "cheat" from my vocabulary. There's really nothing good about cheating in any area of one's life ... including eating. If I choose tasty foods that satisfy, where is the need to cheat?

11. I avoid going to places that *only* serve foods that aren't good for me. (Lots of fast-food restaurants and "ice cream parlors" are off-limits to me.)

12. I take half of my restaurant order home for a future meal. I ask for a take-out or to-go box or container at the time my food is delivered to me at the table.

9. Stop and Go Signs

A good plan should have lots of "stop" moments on the way for you to evaluate your progress as you pursue your wellness goals:

- Have you set goals that are too high? STOP and recalculate. (You aren't going to be able to lose fifty pounds in four weeks.)

- Have you made vows to yourself that are unrealistic? STOP and rethink. (You likely *will* eat a chocolate chip cookie in your future.)

- Have you set out a schedule you had no realistic chance of keeping? STOP and make a new schedule. (You likely aren't going to go to the gym twice a day for the next month, especially if you haven't been to a gym in the last five years.)

- Do you find that you are trying to be like others rather than trying to be the best YOU? STOP and reevaluate. (Nobody is like you and you can't be exactly like anybody else.)

- Do you find yourself criticizing yourself often? STOP it! (There is no benefit in calling yourself names or ridiculing your own failures.)

- Are you making too many excuses? STOP and consider why this might be happening. (You are the only one controlling your time, ultimately, and you are the only one who is holding you accountable for your use of time, ultimately. Rather than make excuses, pursue the goals you *really* want to achieve.)

- Are you blaming failure on others? STOP assigning blame, period. (It shouldn't matter that your workout partner didn't show up.)

- Are you relying on others for motivation? STOP it. (Make *yourself* the foremost person to whom you turn for motivation.)

- Are you bragging about what you are going to do—which is usually a set-up for having to hang your head later for failing? STOP this pattern. (Don't brag about anything— just DO what you say and let your actions speak for themselves.)

- Do you have a "failure mentality"? STOP seeing yourself as a failure waiting to happen. Choose instead to see yourself as a success story that is unfolding!

Looking for the Light to Turn Green. We all love green lights, don't we? That's the time to put your foot on the gas and GO!

You can insert green lights into your Wellness Plan by putting an ACTION STEP next to each goal you identify for your life. When you identity the FIRST step you can and must take to begin your journey toward a goal … you are also identifying the BEST STEP you can take if you get bogged down in your pursuit of a goal. If you get stuck, revisit your goals and pay special attention to the action steps you have assigned to them. That's your clue to turn the lights GREEN.

> The FIRST STEPS you identified as you began your Wellness Plans are very likely the BEST STEP you can take if you get bogged down in your pursuit of a goal.

10. Take on Generational Patterns

As I have traveled the world, I have enjoyed being a "people watcher." Overall, watching other people in action is the least expensive and most enjoyable pastime most people can have!

Not long ago I was in the Los Angeles airport terminal and I observed a father and mother walking toward me, with their two adult children—girls who appeared to be in their early twenties—following close behind. They all looked as if they were struggling to walk the distance of the terminal hall to their gate. The reason was obvious—each person in that family was at *least* 150 pounds overweight! I tried to imagine what the children of these "children" were going to look like. In my mind's eye, they also were severely obese.

A generational problem was clearly in effect, and the sadness for me was not only the fact that all four people struggled to walk four hundred feet before collapsing into the chairs of the waiting area near me, but that I knew there was a significant possibility that neither the mother nor the father of these girls would live to see their grandchildren reach school age, and unless the girls took action, they likely would have a significant difficulty getting pregnant.

Let me encourage you today if you believe you are the "victim" of generational disease, poor eating and exercise patterns, or psychological problems. There IS help available. Ask for it. Seek it out.

You do not need to live like your parents or grandparents lived. You do not need to carry poor health patterns forward into the next generation. You do not need to struggle with the stress, anxiety, fears, discouragement, and depression that one or both of your parents—and perhaps even grandparents—experienced or continue to experience. You can change things, and in doing so, you can alter your own future and the futures of others you love.

11. Not a Number

Most people I know hate being "just a number" in a crowd.

And yet … many people seem to think they ARE a certain "number" on a weight scale, or a certain clothing size. They often use one of these numbers in setting their wellness goals or their weight-loss goals. The true measure to use in setting Wellness Plan goals is how well you *feel*—in other words, how much energy and strength you have.

- Can you get through an entire day without feeling a sinking need for a nap?

- Do you get up in the morning feeling *fatigued*?

- Are you strong enough to do everyday household and yard chores without panting for breath or feeling weak in some part of your body?

If your answer is NO to any of the above … you need to identify changes you need to make to have the energy and strength God wants you to have in order to do the things He has planned for your blessings in this life!

Also ask:

- Do you see your identity as wrapped up in a certain dress size or jacket size?

- Do you believe that thin people are more valuable to God than people who are not thin?

- Do you think you are a "bad" person if you gain a pound during a given week?

Change your perspective! You are NOT a number on a scale or clothing tag.

12. Can or Can't?

There's a famous quote usually attributed to Henry Ford: "If you think you can or can't ... you're right."

People don't usually try to do things they don't think they CAN do.

A life with great possibilities begins with having deep within you the idea of "possibility" for a great life! It truly isn't a matter of what you *can't* do in your life. It is a matter of what you CAN do.

In order to have a can-do attitude you need first of all to take control of your own thoughts and embrace the concept that you can do more, be more, have more, and leave more.

In doing more, you are embracing the idea of accomplishment.

In being more, you are embracing the idea of your unlimited character development.

In having more, you are not only embracing the idea of material acquisition, but also the acquisition of knowledge, or a growing circle of friends, and of having greater and greater influence.

In leaving more, you are embracing the idea of a life marked by generosity and significant "contributions" to others—both individuals and groups. It all starts with what you believe to be POSSIBLE for you.

All lasting change begins inside you, and works its way outward through your words and deeds. A can-do attitude will result in let's-do words, and eventually in ongoing deeds. Along the way, a can-do person exerts *INFLUENCE*, both by what others witness in their lives and by the acts of justice they help implement.

Don't let anybody tell you that you can't do or be something. Prove them wrong!

When faced with what sometimes seems to be an impossible goal or deadline, a friend of mine usually voices these words: "I don't know if can do this … but I don't know that I can't. So, I have to try."

Make that your perspective!

You are given each new morning as your opportunity for a fresh start. Take advantage of it!

---

13. Appreciate the Moment

There's great danger in living in the past … or the future. This seems to be especially true when it comes to pursuit of a Wellness Plan. If you think only of your past, you are likely to become discouraged that you ever allowed yourself to get "out of shape" after earlier years of being "in shape." If you think only of the future, you may become discouraged in those moments when you are making slow progress—you may begin to think, "I'll never get there."

Stay in the present tense. Although your goals AIM you at your future, choose to live in the NOW moments ... and to appreciate them!

Recently while I was on a business getaway with my wife, we were both struck by the beauty of our surroundings—the mountains, waterfalls, and sunshine all combined to give us an indescribable joy and inner peace. We began to talk about the number of places we each had visited that we recalled as being very beautiful, even to the point of "enchantment." We also commented on the fact that we each had no doubt been in places of great beauty that we had failed to appreciate. We had been too preoccupied with other tasks to see what was all around us.

I encourage people periodically to:

- Stop and ask the question, "Where am I?" The answer may seem to be obvious at first, but think about the question further. Don't just "name" where you are, but seek to describe it. What does your current location look like, smell like, feel like, sound like, and so forth.

- Ask, "What am I doing?" What has brought you to this place ... what do you anticipate doing while you are here ... what have you planned or left unplanned? How do you intend to use your time in the place where you are?

- Ask, "How do I feel?" Dig deep for your response. Describe the emotions you are experiencing. Say aloud the predominant feeling you have.

The asking and answering of these three questions can help you enjoy a moment to the max and not "miss" the beauty or pleasure that God is providing for you day by day, experience by experience.

It's also great rehearsal for your five-minute mini-vacations! The more you take in beautiful and meaningful moments, the easier it will be to recall them and use them as you anticipate and plan for bright moments in your future.

14. Detoxification

Detoxing—or doing one's best to detoxify one's body, mind, or spirit—is a popular concept in health-related literature these days. Do you have a good definition for this concept?

Many associate the word "detoxification" with laxatives or cathartics that expel unwanted waste products from the body. The greater reality is that the body has a variety of systems to keep itself detoxed, which includes the elimination of all substances that are not beneficial to the functioning of cells and body organs.

The four main organs of detoxification within the human body are:

1. The skin—the largest organ of detoxification

2. The liver

3. The kidneys

4. The bowels (lower intestines and colon)

Some consider the lungs to be involved in detoxification. The process in the lungs is one of expelling toxins, but not necessarily changing them or completely eliminating them. Air pollutants of many kinds—including self-induced pollutants related to tobacco use—are taken into the lungs and healthy lungs will act almost immediately to *expelling* as much of the toxin as possible. What cannot be expelled, however, tends to accumulate in the cells of the lungs (often as a tar-like substance), or makes its way into the bloodstream.

When we consume toxins in our food, the way for those toxins to make their way out of the body is through the liver, kidneys, and bowels. Too much toxin creates an overload on these systems, which is often experienced as fatigue, body aches and pains, slow mental processing, heart palpitations, gut dysfunctions, or weight increase.

The best way to address the negative impact of toxins is this: AVOID THEM:

- Decrease the number of foods that cause ill effects. This includes avoiding all trans fats and limiting foods high in saturated fats. These fats break down into toxins. Avoid eating vegetables that have been sprayed with pesticides or are coated in wax.

- Stop smoking cigarettes, drinking alcohol, and using drugs. Many over-the-counter medications also can become toxic in the body.

- See exercise as your friend in toxin reduction. The skin eliminates waste products through perspiration. A simple rapid walk on a park path can help your body clear itself of metabolic pollutants!

- Drink plenty of water to flush toxins out of your system, and to dilute their impact on the organs responsible for elimination. Water improves perspiration rates, and helps keep the kidneys, liver, and bowels functioning smoothly.

Toxins are frequently stored as fatty molecules that do not mix well in water. It is part of the function of the gut, liver, and kidneys to transform fat-soluble substances into water-soluble molecules for excretion. Sufficient water in the system is essential for this to happen!

15. Practical Try-Them Tips

Below are six very practical tips related to food and eating that I routinely present to my clients:

1. Keep temptation out of your cupboards. Most people recognize that it is helpful to clear out their cupboards and shelves at the start of a new eating regimen. But often, the "bad stuff" creeps back into the kitchen. Don't leave temptation lying around. Clear out all sugar snacks and drinks from your cupboards at home, and also from your private food stash at work (perhaps that section of your filing cabinet that is exclusively for your use only!).

Go on a search-and-destroy mission for sugar and hydrogenated oils and any items that have saturated fats.

2. Never reward your weight-loss achievements with food. Instead, reward yourself with a makeover, a photo shoot of the "new you," new clothes, a vacation to the beach, or a weekend of hiking a favorite or famous trail.

3. Read food labels and learn the code words. ALERT! Food packagers rarely use the word SUGAR on their labels. What you will find are the words or phrases "high fructose corn syrup," "sucrose," "fructose," or the name or chemical compound of an artificial sweetener (none of which have good nutritional value). Know what you are reading! And if you can't pronounce an ingredient on a food label, don't put that product into your shopping cart!

4. Divide your dinner plate in half ... visually. On the one side put a protein source—a piece of lean range-fed beef, a chicken breast without the skin, a piece of turkey breast, or a piece of fish. On the other half, put low-glycemic-index carbohydrates (fruits and vegetables).

5. If you do not own a Glycemic Index chart, you can purchase one for just a couple of dollars. Become familiar with the vegetables and fruits that are "low glycemic" and avoid the starches that are high on the glycemic scale (mostly items such as potatoes, rice, pasta, breads, and grains in general).

6. Serve your evening meal on a luncheon-sized plate. Fill the plate but have only one plateful of food for your meal. The visual effect will send a signal to your brain of generosity! You might also try eating with a smaller fork—perhaps one that is normally used for seafood.

16. Exercise Is a GOOD Word

If you have come to believe that exercise is a "negative" concept, think again.

Exercise is the foremost means of keeping blood pressure in the right range, promoting a person's balance and flexibility, keeping a person's weight in the right range, and helping control blood chemistry factors.

Exercise is a prime way to improve immunity and in many cases, keep a person motivated when it comes to weight control. Exercise also helps cleanse your body of toxins through perspiration.

Your body was designed for movement. The purpose of your muscles, bones, ligament, and tendons is so you can MOVE with a significant degree of strength, endurance, and flexibility. You can lose strength and flexibility if you don't keep moving. You also can invite more disease and hormonal imbalance if you stop moving.

The lymph system in your body—so vital to immunity—only functions when the body is in MOTION?

So ...

Keep moving!

If you fail temporarily in your exercise goals, start again. Forgive yourself and make a new commitment to do something that is VERY GOOD for you.

If you experience pain while you are exercise, take that as a signal to stop and rest. There is very little advantage in trying to "push through the pain." Find the reason for your pain before you start exercising again. Let me assure you of this, pain is not a sign that you should stop exercising forever ... only temporarily!

Work with a trainer or physical therapist to rehabilitate your body after an injury. If you continue to try to exercise with a broken bone, torn ligament or tendon, ruptured disc, or pulled muscle, you will only delay your pursuit of better fitness and may become so discouraged that you quit exercising altogether. Don't let it happen!

You are never too old for exercise. Studies have shown that even people in nursing homes who were invited to classes where they were taught very minimal forms of "movement" showed *some* improvement in all areas of both their physical and emotional health!

Start talking positively about *exercise*. It is a good word!

You Have My Permission ...

You have my permission to use any of the sixteen essays in this section of the book as the outline or text for a presentation YOU might give about wellness.

The more you TALK about wellness, the more you will be reinforcing the concepts of wellness to your own mind and heart.

And the more you will be encouraging greater health and wholeness to others whom you love or value.

Information about wellness can nearly always be linked to biblical principles if you are asked to give a "devotional" to a Bible-study or church-fellowship group. Information about wellness always can be presented to a community-service club or sports club, especially if the organization is sponsoring or participating in a charity run/walk or specific game or athletic event.

And if you need more ideas to consider for such a presentation … there are additional "nuggets" in the chapter between Phase 2 and Phase 3!

6

NEXT STEPS
PHASE 2

A FRIEND RECENTLY TOLD ME that after her very first driving lesson with her father—an event that occurred when she was barely fifteen—she announced to her father, "This is a piece of cake. Can I borrow the car this Saturday night?"

Her father replied quickly, "Only in your dreams."

When she told me that story I said with a little laugh, "Surely you weren't serious,"

She answered, "Oh, I was very serious. But ... we had been driving through nearby agricultural fields. I hadn't been out on the freeway yet!"

Are you ready to move on to Phase 2? *Are you sure?*

I recommend that a person stay with the goals and activities associated with Phase 1 of their Wellness Plan for a full month before setting out to tackle the behaviors identified in Phase 2.

That gives time for problem areas to surface, and for a person to solidify a FRESH COMMITMENT to the pursuit of additional goals.

All of the activities in Phase 2 are built upon those in Phase 1.

The activities in Phase 2 are built upon those in Phase 1. Continue to do those things you began in Phase 1.

NEXT STEPS —

PHYSICAL

- Engage in 15 minutes of cardio exercise 4x a week
- Do resistance (weight) training 2x a week
- Have 5 servings of vegetables a day
- Avoid all sugar and alcohol
- Replace dairy milk with almond or coconut milk
- Maintain a health log
- Wean yourself off caffeine
- Eliminate bread and starchy carbs
- Eliminate all fried or fatty foods

EMOTIONAL

- Make a budget (monthly)
- Set at least 3 appointments with friends for relationship building
- Spend at least 10 minutes a day in meaningful conversation with your spouse and with each child who lives in your home
- List as part of your personal journal the names of people you will seek out to compliment or affirm (in person or in writing)

Set Goals + Consolidate and Balance + Reset Goals +

A person must continue to do those things that they have started in Phase 1. In some cases, more time or greater quantity is recommended, but previous behaviors are never entirely set aside. Don't lose sight of that principle!

If a suggestion on these pages involves more time or a greater quantity, make that adjustment.

PHASE 2

INTELLECTUAL

- Turn off junk media and limit your "news" watching to no more than 30 minutes a day
- List and define your own values in your personal journal
- Detox your thought life
- Develop the habit of planning your next day the night before
- Set aside part of your journal for writing new "ideas" or opinion statements that are motivational to you—discover what truly motivates YOU

SPIRITUAL

- Begin a THANKS log and add 5 entries to it each day
- Begin a PRAISE log and add at least one entry to it each day
- Clear your heart at the end of of each day (asking God for forgiveness, direction, and a night of sweet sleep)

Get Counseling if you need it + Keep a Personal Journal

Notes about the PHYSICAL Dimension of Phase 2

1. Increase your cardio activity.

Cardio exercises are also called "aerobic" exercises. I prefer the term cardio because not all so-called aerobic exercise is done at a level that makes it truly *aerobic*.

A true aerobic exercise is one that elevates the heart rate on a continual basis and keeps it elevated over a period of time. The elevated heart rate is ideally continued for at least ten minutes.

There are many physically stressful activities that are NOT true aerobic exercises—such as tennis, weight training, racquetball, short sprint racing, and some stationary bike "spinning." The reason is that these exercises do not produce a CONSISTENT elevation in heart rate, only "spurts" of elevated numbers.

To evaluate your own aerobic exercise, you need to know your resting heart rate (beats per minute) when you are sitting in a chair, and then have a heart rate monitor or use a stopwatch during an exercise period to take your pulse while you are exercising at what you consider to be a maximum level of effort.

What should be your "maximum heart rate"? Subtract your age from 220. If a person is fifty years old, 220 minus 50 is 170. That's a maximum heart rate for the person but it is not the ideal heart rate for optimized aerobic activity. The aerobic heart rate desired is 65 percent to 85 percent of the maximum heart rate. For the fifty-year-old, that would be 110 to 144 beats per minutes.

A leisurely stroll through the park or on a treadmill will not accomplish this mission. Neither will slow pedaling on a stationary bicycle. Does this mean that you should not do exercises unless you reach true aerobic output? Not at all. Start where you can and do as much as you can. Recognize along the way that you may not truly be doing *aerobic* exercising, but also applaud yourself for being on your way toward that goal.

2. Do resistance or strength training.

Women have frequently said to me, "Dr. Mark, I don't want to lift weights" and when I ask, "Why not?" they reply, "I don't want to look like a man." If you have that concern, let me quickly assure you that you will NOT look like a man if you use weights to tone up your muscles. For one thing, women do not have the necessary structure in their bodies to build "bulked up" muscle. And for another thing, the types of exercises this plan recommends are not the ones used for "heavy weight training." The exercises are for the growth of LEAN muscle (which is critical to increased metabolism and fat burning), and to stimulate increased density of the bones (more calcium, more stability, and a less likelihood of osteoporosis).

Personalize Your Plan. Begin your resistance training by visiting with a professional trainer, perhaps someone at a gym where you go to swim or walk an indoor track. Every person's needs are different and a trainer can help you focus on areas of your body that provide maximum help for your heart muscle and other muscle groups.

Exercise is not a one-type-fits-all proposition. Customize your exercise plan for YOUR body and your lifestyle.

The Basic Process of Building Lean Muscle. It may help you to know that "lean muscle mass" is built by a threefold process of 1) tearing down, 2) resting and recovery, and 3) rebuilding. When a person lifts weights, muscle tissue is slightly broken down (or slightly torn apart). During rest or recovery periods, this process turns into one of rebuilding. What happens in rebuilding is this: the body does not just restore the muscle back to its previous condition, but it actually rebuilds muscle tissue that is STRONGER than before. This means that the next time the body is asked to lift the same amount of weight, it finds it easier to do so. Over time, weight needs to be increased for the tearing down, rest and recovery, and rebuilding process to continue to produce stronger and stronger muscle tissue.

Adding weight to an exercise is one way of increasing the effectiveness of strength training. Another way is to increase the exercise intensity by shortening the rest period between sets. And yet another way is to perform more repetitions.

You will be wise to make these adjustments with the help of a trainer. Lessening the time between sets or performing more repetitions may mean *decreasing* the weight you have been lifting. Over time, that weight can be increased.

There are also variations in the type of exercise a person can do to exercise more muscle groups more effectively. For example, a flat bench press might be exchanged for an incline bench press, or a flat bench press might be exchanged for a flat dumbbell press. Again, work with a trainer.

If it sounds a little as if you are trying to trick your own muscles … well, you are! You are mixing up the routine so that you are continually challenging your own muscle tissue to become stronger.

Prepare yourself for setbacks. You will find that some weeks you don't make your goal. Don't beat yourself up about that. Just resolve to get back into the rhythm of what you desire to do to reach the goal you desire to achieve. Remind yourself of your GOAL, and let the accomplishment of it motivate you.

A Good Resistance (Strength) Training Protocol:
2–3 days a week do these exercises:

- Squats/Leg Press — 5 sets of 10–12 repetitions
- Bench Press — 4 sets of 10–12 reps
- Lat Pull Downs (to the front) — 5 sets of 10–12 reps

Rest about 90 seconds between sets, and rest at least one day before repeating this workout. (In other words, do not do this protocol on consecutive days.) For a person who is accustomed to working out in a gym, this may seem like a very simple, basic routine, but I assure you that if you give yourself proper rest between workouts, the workout will be very effective.

Some people believe that resistance or weight exercises are only for the upper body—they erroneously think that jogging or running will *strengthen* leg muscles. Not so! Jogging and running are aerobic activities that strengthen the heart, lungs, and respiratory system. To strengthen the lower body, exercises need to be done with weights that build up leg and hip muscles. To strengthen the arms, flexibility exercises are nearly always the most beneficial. Balanced physiques are always the goal.

Leg, back, and chest muscles are larger than arm muscles and therefore, the training of arm muscles requires fewer reps and fewer sets. Here are two workouts for arm muscles:

Workout #1 for Arms

Alternate these two:
- Machine Triceps pushdowns — 3 sets (10, 8, 6 reps)
- Dumbbell biceps curls — 3 sets (10, 8, 6 reps)

Alternate these two:
- Triceps kick backs — 2 sets (10, 8 reps)
- Hammer curls (dumbbells) — 2 sets (10, 8 reps)

Workout #2 for Arms

Alternate these two:
- Dips — 4 sets (10, 10, 10)
- Barbell curls — 4 sets (10, 10, 10)

Keep track of the weights you are using and gradually increase weight when you find that you can complete a set with the identified reps *with ease*.

3. Eat more vegetables (for antioxidant protection).

Eat your vegetable and limited fruit portions in a "fresh" and "whole food" state if possible (not in juice or frozen). If you have two servings at lunch, two at dinner, and add berries or greens to a morning protein drink ... that will be five servings a day!

4. Avoid all sugar and alcohol.

A man once said to me, "I'm all for avoiding sugar—you've convinced me about that ... but give up all alcohol?"

I replied, "Alcoholic beverages are mostly sugar."

He gulped and said a simple, "OK."

Every time I hear on the media a so-called "medical report" that advocates the acceptability of one to two drinks of alcohol a day as good for a person's health ... I cringe. In the course of my work for more than two decades in the wellness industry, I have seen more than one of my colleagues and friends overtaken by the effects of alcohol consumption. Alcohol is a powerful addictive chemical that can lead one very quickly toward a slow, torturous death.

Not everybody processes alcohol in the same way, but I can guarantee you this: alcohol moves very quickly through the body. It enters the bloodstream without being metabolized in the stomach—most alcohol consumed is in the blood system within five minutes after intake. Within thirty to ninety minutes, the alcohol in a person's bloodstream is at the highest level. If a person is drinking alcohol at a rate faster than the liver can break it down, the alcohol causes damage to the liver. Unprocessed alcohol then moves through the brain and the body to damage cells at a high rate. Any person who drinks even one glass of an alcoholic beverage should do so *very slowly*.

When a prediabetic person consumes alcohol, he or she is susceptible to hypoglycemia, which is an abnormally low blood glucose level. Hypoglycemia can cause seizures, unconsciousness, and in some cases, brain damage or death.

Nearly all alcoholic beverages are *very high* in calories! At the same time, they are very low in nutritional value. If you insist on having a drink, select an alcoholic beverage that is low in alcohol content and sugar, such as a spritzer. Mix the drink with a sugar free substance such as tonic water or club soda.

Never consume alcohol on an empty stomach.

Much has been said about the value of red wine. The beneficial substance in red wine is resveratrol—and this can be taken in a capsule of red-wine extract for all the benefits, at a fraction of the cost, and without the negative effects of alcohol!

If a person is drinking alcohol and eating at the same time, the body will metabolize the alcohol first and store the food as fat. The "caloric energy" from alcohol is NEVER stored – the body perceives that alcohol is a poison and it seeks to process it and eliminate it as quickly as possible. The improperly metabolized food is absorbed by the body and stored *without* the benefit of the food's minerals and vitamins ever being used.

Too much alcohol nearly always leads to insulin resistance and increased weight loss, with almost a direct line to diabetes.

What about sugar substitutes? Most "artificial sweeteners" are a chemical nightmare and should be avoided. Stevia leaf or Truvia sweeteners (plant based) are better for you than refined sugar or artificial sweeteners. If you are served a dessert and don't see any way to refuse it without being considered grossly impolite, eat only a few bites (no more than half a portion).

5. Find a dairy substitute you like.

I personally have come to *prefer* coconut milk or almond milk over so-called regular milk.

Keep in mind that dairy products include cheese, cottage cheese, yogurt, and ice cream. Ice creams and yogurts are often loaded with sugar.

And … regular cow's milk is loaded with lactose, which is *sugar*. Many people are lactose-intolerant. Cow's milk is also high in fat unless you buy *nonfat* products.

Goat cheese is better than cheese made from cow's milk. Hard cheeses, such as parmesan, are better than most soft cheeses when it comes to fat content.

6. Keep a health log.

This documentation may be part of what you write in your personal journal, or it may be a separate accounting of what you eat and how you exercise.

In completing a basic health log:

- Write down *everything* you eat, including condiments. A complete listing of all foods can help you isolate unrecognized food allergies (if you have them), and if you will add how *much* of a particular food you consume, you can come close to determining how many calories you are eating at every meal.

- Estimate your total calorie intake every day.

- Write down what type of exercise you do, and the duration or number of reps.

- If you are a diabetic or pre-diabetic, record your fasting glucose number every morning.

You may want to weigh yourself daily, or not. Some people find that a daily "accounting" keeps them more cautious when it comes to overeating opportunities. Other people find the periodic fluctuations in water weight to be discouraging. Do what works best for you.

Make notes in your health log about how you "feel"—energetic, sluggish, positive, negative, exhausted, enthusiastic, and so forth. Note if you are ill (a cold, flu) or are struggling with a chronic ailment (such as constipation).

As much as possible, plan your meals in advance of eating them. You can do this weekly, or perhaps for every three to four days in advance. This will help you make a grocery list—and if you stick to the list, you'll help yourself when it comes to potential binge buying and later, binge eating.

7. Wean yourself off caffeine.
8. Eliminate bread and starchy carbs.
9. Eliminate all fried or fatty foods.

Let's take these three together.

Through the years, I have developed three "challenges" that I give to various clients at various times.

Challenge #1: Deal with the Big Three

Both bread and dairy products break down into *sugars* and the three food categories of bread, dairy, and sugar are the greatest contributors to being overweight. Most people have difficulty in giving up bread, sugar, and dairy products all at the same time. I recommend a fourteen-day "weaning" process:

- DAY 1   Eliminate sugar (still eat bread and dairy)
- DAY 2   Eliminate bread (still eat sugar and dairy)
- DAY 3   Eliminate dairy (still eat sugar and bread)
- DAY 4   Eliminate sugar, bread, and dairy TOTALLY
- DAY 5   Eliminate sugar (still eat bread and dairy)
- DAY 6   Eliminate bread (still eat sugar and dairy)
- DAY 7   Eliminate dairy (still eat sugar and bread)
- DAY 8   Eliminate sugar, bread, and dairy TOTALLY
- DAY 9   Eliminate sugar and bread (still eat dairy)
- DAY 10 Eliminate bread and dairy (still eat sugar)

- DAY 11 Eliminate sugar and dairy (still eat bread)

- DAY 12 Eliminate the BIG THREE totally (no sugar, bread, or dairy)

- DAY 13 Have a Mardi Gras day (eat whatever you like)

- DAY 14 Eliminate the BIG THREE totally

Why do this? You will be readjusting your own thinking patterns. This plan has four days of TOTAL elimination of the three food groups that are most damaging to your health.

The plan requires you to be AWARE of what you are putting into your mouth. Awareness is the first real step in making any permanent lifestyle change.

The plan proves to YOU, the foremost critic required to convince, that you CAN do without one, two, or even three food categories.

Challenge #2: Dr. Mark's Insane One-Week Challenge

If you feel pretty positive after dealing with the big three, or if you are feeling pretty good about your overall progress, it may be time for you to accept my Insane One-Week Challenge.

- Day 1 — Avoid all sugar. This is tough but chances are, you've allowed a little sugar to creep back into your diet.

- Day 2 — Avoid sugar and all dairy. If you've been using dairy for part of your protein nutrition, this may be harder than you think.

- Day 3 — Avoid all sugar, dairy, and caffeine.

- Day 4 — avoid all sugar, dairy, caffeine, and alcohol. This won't be any harder than day 3 if you aren't a drinker.

- Day 5 — Avoid all sugar, dairy, caffeine, alcohol, and all processed and packaged foods. Fat burning is likely kicking in!

- Day 6 — Avoid all sugar, dairy, caffeine, alcohol, processed and packaged foods, and gluten. Dig in and get tough!

- Day 7 — Avoid all sugar, dairy, caffeine, alcohol, processed and packaged foods, gluten, and take a thirty-minute brisk walk.

Challenge #3: Drop a "Type" of Food a Week, for Six Weeks.

Another approach to controlling the intake of certain detrimental foods is to drop a "type" of food a week, for six weeks. Many people can do themselves a world of GOOD by eliminating the foods below:

- Fatty cuts of beef and pork

- Stick margarine

- Fried fast foods

- Pastry or other packaged baked goods

- Whole milk dairy products (unless natural, organic, pasture-raised and grass fed)

- Skin from chicken and turkey

Notes about the Emotional Dimension of Phase 2

1. Make a monthly financial budget.

I recommend that you do this with a financial advisor and with your spouse involved in the process. The financial advisor can be an objective voice of reason for you, and having your spouse on board with the budgeting process is always a good idea.

Overall, wellness is a process of stewardship—of taking care of your total life in the best possible way. This concept of stewardship applies to your physical health, as well as to the acquisition, care, and giving of material items. All things come to you from God. Ultimately, all things belong to Him. You are a manager, not the boss.

2. Appointments with friends (nurture relationships).

Don't wait until a friend moves away or dies to wish you had spent more time with the person.

Make friends with people of many ages—from elderly to young. Spend time listening to their experiences, insights, and dreams (even the elderly often have dreams and goals!). Enjoy the blessing of a mutually caring, mutually beneficial *friendship*.

3. Have meaningful conversations.

So much of daily "talk" is about tasks, chores, or appointments. Take time every day in one-to-one conversation with your spouse, and with each child living in your home. Talk about what the *other* person wants to talk about. (You'll get your chance, especially if you give the other person their chance first!)

Talk as much as possible about things that really *matter* ... which tend to be things that are likely to matter a year from now.

4. Target people to compliment or applaud.

Choose to be an encourager. There are so few of them in our world today. Don't overlook the people you live with or see often, thinking, *oh, they know I value them.* Tell them. Nobody ever gets tired of hearing the words "I love you" or "I appreciate you!"

Notes about the Intellectual Dimension of Phase 2

1. Detox your intake of information.

We often limit our understanding of the process called "detoxification." There are forms of detoxification that are related to a person's emotional and mental life!

I recently told a group something I had not *planned* to say, but later, I was very glad I said it. "There is a ton of toxic information out there."

Much of the information that is toxic to us is outright lies or false. Unfortunately, those who tout lies often do so with such boldness that the listener or reader assumes that only the truth could be stated with such conviction or forcefulness. Not so!

A significant amount of toxic information is presented in

speculation. Listen closely to nightly newscasts, and especially to commentary and "talk-show" programs. There are times when I've taken notes and come to the realization that about seventy percent of what I was "told" was sheer speculation—things were "alleged," "according to a supposed authority," a prediction was made about the near or long-range future that could not be anything BUT speculation, or a report was heavily punctuated with "opinions" that were given merit as if they were universal truth.

Be careful what you listen to. Be even more careful about what you believe.

I am especially suspicious of information that presents products with a general impression that a specific substance can "change your life." Maybe a little, but rarely a lot. There are no magic bullets, and no quick fixes. Everything changes us in some way—but in many cases, the purchase of a life-changing product only changes the amount of money in the person's bank account or wallet.

This is also true for products and plans that promise to significantly alter a person's life— within a set time frame—be it their health, weight, financial portfolio, or love life. Claims are often made for obvious change or results in "the next two weeks," or "within thirty days," or "by summer" (which might be sixty days away). These claims are often highly improbable, if not impossible!

How can you detox your intellectual life?

- Ask questions, And continue to ask them.

- Get second opinions. And sometimes a third or fourth opinion.

- Avoid disaster theories and doomsday reports. The "end" will come but you can't predict the day nor hour. And until that end point comes, you have a responsibility to live a life of faith, confidence, and positive pursuits.

- Voice opinions sparingly. You may not know what you don't know.

- Listen to opinions from others but be slow to agree. Don't jump on any crusader bandwagon solely on the basis of a leader's personal charm or force of personality.

- Engage in open and direct conversations as much as you can do so. Don't fall into the traps of continual "political correctness" or "prevailing opinion." Sometimes political correctness is NOT correct and a so-called prevailing opinion is not truly PREVAILING!

- Continue learning about things that interest you. Don't ever think you know it all—even in your area of expertise or specialty. There may be a legitimate new discovery or new study that can impact your effectiveness and the quality of your life and work.

- Recognize always that quality products cost more than inferior products. Be wise in what you buy—whether it is "tuition," a service, a product, or advice.

2. Identify your core values.

We all have values, although most people don't often take time to identify their values. Choose to be intentional in doing this. Reflect on what you think and believe. Two good questions to ask are:

- How committed am I to the TRUTH?
- What DON'T I want to live without?

Honest answers can be highly self-revealing!

3. Plan your day the night before.

Make a list of "things to do" before you go to sleep at night. Prioritize the list. That way when you get up in the morning, you already have a focus for your day!

4. Discover what motivates you.

I once had a client who worked in the world of high finance. He told me that he was motivated to develop a Wellness Plan because he "couldn't afford to get sick." He saw wellness as a real investment with real dollar value. I have since used his approach in my wellness counseling, especially with clients who are in the brokerage, banking, or financial counseling industries.

This man pointed out to me the costs of four common surgical procedures, each of which had been experienced by one of his parents or an extended family member:

- Heart surgery — $100,000
- Gastric bypass — $ 22,000

- Liposuction — $ 3,000
- Knee replacement — $ 50,000

And that's assuming there are no complications or follow-up infections and treatment required.

I am not devaluing the cost of these procedures. Physicians should not be expected to work for free and each of these procedures requires a medical *team*. What I am saying is that you might find a very real, practical, financial ADVANTAGE in living in a way that greatly reduces your ever needing heart surgery, gastric bypass, liposuction, or a knee replacement.

Find Your Why. I once had another client with a very different perceived need for greater wellness.

His opening line in our first meeting was this: "I need your help … I don't want to die."

I gulped. The truth is, every person on the planet is going to *die* … someday. I didn't know what this man was facing or why he was making that statement. I could see with my eyes that he was probably fifty to seventy pounds overweight, and his skin and complexion were sallow. I could hear discouragement in his voice and could also see it in his body language. I asked as gently and politely as I could, "Are you dealing with a terminal diagnosis?"

He gave a faint smile and said, "Sorta. The doctor told me that if I didn't make some major changes in my health habits, I would not live to dance at my daughter's wedding."

"And when is that wedding?" I asked.

He smiled a little bigger. "She's eight years old."

"Oh, good," I said with a big sigh of relief. "We have some time. Let's get busy on your wellness plan so you can enjoy *lots* of happy events between now and then, and then, even happier times after the wedding."

We mapped out a plan and he began to work the plan.

Within six months, he had lost forty pounds, and by the end of the first year, he had lost eighty pounds and was well within an appropriate BMI range. He had started working out—walking and lifting light weights—and he was looking more fit. He had changed his eating patterns, and the result was a healthier glow to his skin. All of these positive and visible changes had boosted his self-confidence. He had become more active in his synagogue and had also become more active in a community-service club to which he belonged. He admitted to me that his relationship with his wife had led them to take a "second honeymoon." And his daughter had told him, "Daddy, I am so proud that you are my dad. There are a lot of girls at my school who aren't as lucky as I am."

I couldn't keep myself from saying, "Luck had nothing to do with it. Hard work and a commitment to changing your daily habits brought you to this point." And then I quickly added, "Let's get you on a maintenance plan so you can keep this level of wellness. You still have a lot of years to go before that wedding."

He replied, "Oh, didn't I tell you? My wife is pregnant. We

need to add about twenty more years, at least, to my Wellness Plan!"

I was grateful that this man had found his WHY for pursuing a Wellness Plan, and that it was a happy WHY. Many people don't have a clear motivating PURPOSE for wanting wellness.

Wellness isn't just a nice idea. It is the BEST idea. It includes a person's highest desires for all that is good in life: spiritual depth, emotional blessings, intellectual vibrancy, and physical energy and strength.

Notes about the Spiritual Dimension of Phase 2

1. Create a "thanks" list.

I seem to spend a great deal of time in airport lounges, but I am rarely bored. Some of these times are *very* interesting.

One day I was in eye and earshot of a young father, perhaps 35 years old, who was with his son, about age 8. They sat down next to an older gentleman who was wearing a "Vietnam Veteran" cap, and who seemed to have just returned from a meeting or reunion of fellow veterans. The father entered into a conversation with the man, and in the course of the conversation asked the man to recount some of his military experiences for his son. The veteran spoke of the fear, bloodshed, friendship, and loss he had experience during his time of military service. He told about being wounded, and how painful it had been to return home to find that many people had little appreciation for the time and sacrifice he had given. The young boy asked him, "Was it worth it?"

The older gentleman answered, "Yes, I would do it all again."

The young boy spontaneously moved to the older gentleman and gave him a hug and said, "Thank you." As their flight was called and they prepared to board, the father shook the man's hand and said, "Thank you for your service. And thank you for what you just gave to my son."

I then heard the woman sitting next to the veteran—I hadn't really paid any attention to her before that time—say to the man, "Thank you, dear, for your words to that man and his boy. I was touched by what you said. I am so grateful that God brought you home from the war so I could marry you and be the mother of your children."

He replied, "And I'm grateful, too!"

I thought to myself, *There's more gratitude within ten feet of me than I have experienced during this entire business trip!* I was feeling deep gratitude in ME, for this man's service, his willingness to share his experience, the boy's hug, the father's handshake, the wife's affirmation, and for my opportunity to witness it all and now share it with you. I readily admit I also felt gratitude welling up in me that I am an American, and that most of my fellow Americans believe firmly in freedom and the privilege of helping other people attain it.

Gratitude isn't just for "thanksgiving day." Gratitude should be the very attitude that permeates ALL of our days.

And … gratitude is meant to be EXPRESSED, not just felt.

Take time today to VOICE your gratitude to someone for their contribution to your life—perhaps their good service in waiting on you at lunch, their steadfast love as your spouse or parent or child, their time spent in helping you, their skill rendered in keeping your yard immaculate … their patient teaching of your child to play the trumpet … . there are a thousand people you might thank and ten thousand reasons to give thanks!

Take time this week to WRITE a note of appreciation to someone. It can be a simple one-liner in an email, but it is even more meaningful if a thank you comes in handwritten form through the mail. "Thanks for speaking up on my behalf" … "thank you for your gift—it means a lot" … "thank your for your prayers during this difficult time" … "thank you for your help in raising funds for this cause that means so much to all of us." You don't need to write a world-class essay. Just taking the time and saying the words THANK YOU can make a positive difference in a person's life.

A word of gratitude warms two hearts—
your heart, and the heart of the person who
hears you say "I appreciate you."

---

2. Make a praise list.

We tend to thank people—and God—for what they have done,

past or present, usually in a concrete way that impacts us personally. We tend to offer praise for WHO a person is, and the demonstration of their character.

If you want to be a "superstar" in the world of thank-you notes, include an affirmative word of praise as you express your thanks. Let the person know what you believe about their nature, character, and integrity. You'll make their day, perhaps even their month or year.

3. Close out the day well.

The end of the day, right before bedtime, is a good time to talk to your Creator. I find it an especially meaningful time to:

- Confess what I know were my faults, errors, and sins during the day—in what I thought, said, did, and also in the things that I should have done but didn't do. I find it very cleansing to admit my weakness to God, ask for His forgiveness, and then actively *receive* His forgiveness. (The Bible promises that if we confess our sins to God, He always forgives us freely and fully. See 1 John 1:9.)

- Ask God to guide my steps in the coming day. I actively and intentionally invite God's presence into each appointment that I know I'm facing.

- Ask God to give me a good night's rest. The Bible tells us that God delights in giving His people "sweet sleep"—I take that to mean deep REM levels of sleep and good dreams.

By ending a day well, I nearly always awaken with joy in my heart and an eagerness to discover what God is going to do and how He might use me.

7

NUGGETS OF INFORMATION AND INSPIRATION

(AS YOU MOVE FROM PHASE 2 TO PHASE 3)

AS YOU FIND YOURSELF comfortable with your changes in behavior and with your progress in reaching your Phase 2 goals, step back and do what you did *before* Phase 2. Assess your progress ... revisit and revise your goals if you need to ... and take some time to reflect on how the four dimensions of life are working together to create a greater sense of harmony in your life.

Try to isolate, and perhaps write in your journal about, ways in which your positive changes in the physical dimension have influenced your spiritual, intellectual, and emotional behaviors.

And then do the same for each of the other dimensions. Identify any "synergy" you feel.

Below are more essays presented in the hopes of giving you additional information and inspiration. Enjoy, and again, feel free to retell this information to others.

Nuggets

1. Get Smart about Food

By now in your quest for greater wellness you have been dealing with an eating plan, and perhaps a weight-loss plan, for several weeks, perhaps months. Make sure you know as much as you can about the types of foods you are consuming.

The BIG FOUR lessons that I believe all people need to learn about food and fitness are these:

1. Eating too much sugar leads to obesity, inflammation, metabolic syndrome, diabetes, and heart problems.

2. Reducing or eliminating sugar from our eating pattern can be achieved if we know and use the Glycemic Index (food chart) to monitor and control our carbohydrate intake.

3. Water is the body's greatest need after sufficient air. We need to be drinking at least half of our lean body weight in ounces for good hydration and detoxification.

4. A sedentary lifestyle has been defined by the American Heart Association as a lack of regular exercise at least 3 times a week for three months. A sedentary lifestyle is directly correlated with weight gain (and obesity).

Every person needs the fuel that comes from these three food types:
1. Protein
2. Carbohydrates
3. Fat

The majority of each should come through the foods we eat. Any so-called "diet" plan or eating plan that eliminates one of these three essentials is not going to be healthful for you in the long run.

I had a person once describe to me how you can tell if a food is mostly protein or mostly carbohydrate:

- If the food has or had a "mother," it is probably protein.

- If something came from a tree or out of a plant growing in the soil, it is probably carbohydrate.

Protein. We live in an age in which protein sources are plentiful in our culture. We are especially blessed to have high-quality protein in powder form—these sources often have a complete line-up of the amino acids necessary for cell generation and renewal. Good protein sources are very easy to digest and assimilate.

My favorite choices for protein are grass-fed non-denatured, low-heat-processed whey protein concentrate, miceller casein (a great non-denatured, slowly digested protein source), and egg white or whole egg powder. I also personally like a nondairy pea protein that is created using organic non-GMO yellow peas. (NOTE: whey refers to milk-based protein so the grass-fed stipulation refers to the grass-fed cows from which this milk is taken.)

I alternate my protein sources by day, week, or bimonthly for variety in taste and texture, and also for greater overall protein balance and varying fat intake.

If you see that the number-one protein source in a product you are using is "soy concentrate" or "isolate, sodium caseinate," or "wheat protein (which is basically gluten) … make another choice! Also avoid very low cost whey protein products because they generally come from poor quality sources. As is true for most things in life, you get what you pay for when it comes to quality in protein powders.

How much protein powder should you use? I use this formula: multiply body weight by .6. That is the number of grams of protein needed per day spread throughout 4–5 "mini meals." For a person who weighs 150 pounds, the grams of protein comes to 90.

That's 15–18 grams per serving. This assumes that the person engages mostly in light to moderate activity, perhaps exercising only three times a week.

A person with a high level of activity should multiply their body weight by 1.0 to 1.2. This is the number of grams of protein needed per day spread across 4–5 mini meals.

Carbohydrates. Carbs can usually be evaluated by the Glycemic Index chart, which indicates how rapidly they break down in the digestive process to become fuel. Carbs with a low number on the Glycemic Index are preferred over high-number carbs.

Generally speaking, a person should not each more than a total of 150 carbohydrate grams a day.

Fats. The kind of fat that we need for good health is "essential fatty acids." Take special note of the words essential and acids. This type of fat is not the fat that you see surrounding a steak or floating on top of a bowl of chili.

Avoid excessive saturated fats and all trans fats, including hydrogenated oils and hydrolyzed oil. Check labels. Look for words that indicate oils and if you don't know what they are, take some labels to your nutritionist and find out.

Where do we find essential fatty acids? The best source is fish, and therefore, fish oil. Look for the Omega 3 content on various nutritional supplements.

What about grains? Most breads and other products made from grains should be eaten sparingly or avoided.

If you want to eat grains, I highly recommend seeking out products with sprouted grain—such as Ezekiel Bread, rye kernel, oat bran, or pumpernickel breads. All of these are considered low on the Glycemic Index scale.

I call the "first course" in most restaurants the "great grain giveaway." Many restaurants offer free bread (and sometimes butter to go with it), or chips and salsa as something to keep a customer munching while dinner is being prepared.

What's wrong with this?

Both white bread and corn chips are very high Glycemic-Index foods. In fact, white bread is actually higher on the Glycemic Index than table sugar!

When a person eats bread or chips in large quantity before a meal, the insulin-production system in the body goes into overdrive and a very high percentage of the intake of bread or ships is ushered into the body's cells to be stored as FAT.

Bread and chips are not only bad for a weight-loss plan, they are bad for the maintenance of even blood-sugar levels!

Think "Eating Plan." I prefer the phrase EATING PLAN to the word "diet."

If weight loss is part of your health goals, then you will want to weigh yourself periodically. However, having sufficient energy and strength is a far better goal than setting an "ideal number" that you hope to see on a scale.

In some cases, weight loss is not healthy—especially if it involves malnutrition, a severe or rapid loss of lean muscle tissue, or increases your heart rate artificially. Those who "starve" themselves as they lose weight rarely keep the weight off.

The best weight-loss plans begin and end with this principle:

Eat what is good for your body.

That one principle covers both WHAT to eat and how much

of it to EAT. And, if you add the principle of eating small amounts of nutritionally good foods at regular intervals throughout a day, you will find it easier to stick to eating "right."

Gradual Change Is Best. If you are developing a new way of eating to put yourself into alignment with your Wellness Plan goals, make the changes *gradually*.

You'll find it easier and your mind and body will eventually get into sync about what satisfies. In many ways, the start of a nutrition-based eating plan is the start of "retraining" for your taste buds. Over time, you will discover the REAL taste of certain foods. When people eat foods that are laced with lots of chemical additives and fillers, they become addicted to the taste of fat and sugar, whether they know it or not. When fat and sugar are eliminated, there can be initial feelings of dissatisfaction. But … over time … the "real" taste of food comes through and people often feel highly motivated at the idea of discovering what a truly ripe piece of fruit or a lightly steamed vegetable tastes like! (You may think you know … but do you *really?*)

Balance and Quality. I cannot overemphasize the importance of these two words to a Wellness Plan. When it comes to eating, you must have a *balanced* intake of protein, carbohydrates, and essential fatty acids.

You also are wise to choose the highest quality products and foods in each of the three main categories. When it comes to good nutrition, you really do get what you pay for—don't short-change yourself when it comes to QUALITY ingredients and products.

2. Seek to Become Great

I overheard a child ask one day, "How does a person get to be great?" He had heard about a certain hero in our nation's history and the man had repeatedly been described as a "great man." He wanted to know what it took to win that adjective.

I thought about the question and decided that if anyone ever asked it of me, I would give these three words:

1. **Commitment.** A great person is a person who is committed to doing the right things and doesn't back off that commitment. If he makes a vow, he keeps it. If he gives his word, he is true to it.

2. **Consistency.** Great people have a character that is predictable. The person who displays consistency will find that other people trust their word and follow their lead.

3. **Companionship.** Great people align themselves with people who aspire to do the right things and live with integrity. They choose their friends and associations carefully. You *will* become like the people with whom you spend the most time.

I learned many years ago about the key differences between eagles and vultures, both of which are fierce predators.

Eagles soar above the storms. They build their nests at the top of mountains, and from this vantage point, they are not only safer than most creatures, but they have a panoramic view of the world that allows them to make the most of every opportunity. They have a reputation as a species for nobility and are generally admired.

Vultures hide in the crags of rocks. They are victims of "waiting out storms" rather than rising above them. They very often eat what others consider to be leftovers or spoiled foods (including carnage of prey killed by other predators). They have no reputation for nobility, only of being creatures that are generally despised.

Are you an eagle or vulture? Who are you hanging out with?

3. Six Provocative Questions

Throughout your life, continue to ask yourself provocative questions or to think about provocative statements. Here are several I offer for your consideration:

- Sacks of sugar coming from the Caribbean were once labeled clearly with skull and crossbones emblems indicating "poison!" Sugar is and was toxic and it feeds cancer. Why did we ever allow so much of it into our food?

- Type II diabetes is man-made. We create it by over-ingesting sugars and sugar-like substances. Why do we allow this to happen?

- Where did we get the idea of "fast food"? God did not make fast food.

- Why do we think we have the right to genetically modify foods? Are we trying to play God?

- How much food is *enough*?

- If healthcare is improving, why are we seeing more and more cancer centers?

4. Expanding Your Emotional Quotient

Although the jury of educational researchers is still "out" when it comes to whether a person can expand his or her "intelligence quotient," most people do believe it is possible to expand one's "emotional quotient" (EQ). We can learn to change our emotional responses, and to diversify them to better fit circumstances.

We can *decide* that certain things we have never thought of as "fun" are actually enjoyable! We can change both attitude and perception.

Many of the disciplines associated with food management and exercise are not considered fun by many people. A perspective of dread, loathing, or discouragement is not helpful, however. In fact, it is counterproductive. I am not going to ask you to think of dieting or exercise as FUN, but I can tell you this—people who successfully diet and routinely exercise tend to HAVE more fun in life and over time; they often do think of a good-for-you gourmet meal (high on good taste and texture, void of fatty sauces) or a good workout as a pleasurable experience.

Change your thinking. It's the biggest challenge when it comes to adopting good nutritional and fitness habits. It is also helpful in this way: You do not need to internalize the STRESS that can come by resisting, avoiding, hating, or otherwise thinking negatively about good nutrition or exercise. If you dwell on the fact that you "gotta eat right" or "must eat less" or "must get to the gym" or "just have to run," you are going to add additional stress to your life and that is going to be counterproductive—at least to a degree. The easiest thing to do is to say:

"Thank God I can make good choices and still have good enough health and flexibility to MOVE my body."

And then pursue that blessing!

Four Main Emotional Lessons to Learn. I am a strong advocate for the need to teach, and subsequently LEARN, the four emotional lessons below.

1. **Debt.** Spending more than you make and living "beyond" your means leads to debt, and debt deprives a person of freedom and spontaneity. It leads to competition ("keeping up with the neighbors") and causes more family and marital problems than any other relational issue. Debt also can lower a person's sense of self-esteem or self-value, and keep a person from engaging freely in charitable projects or ministries.

2. **Control Issues.** Attempting to change or control others is rarely beneficial—either to you or to the other person. In the end, the only person who can make a lasting

change is the person himself or herself—and in the vast majority of cases, true change only happens when the person invites God to be part of the change process. Trying to make another person change or conform to your design is not only futile, therefore, but it can seriously zap your emotional stability, energy levels, and time. Playing "God" is not a role you were designed to play in life.

3. **Conflict and Anger.** Conflict should be *mostly* avoided. There are times when a person must speak up or take action to ensure the safety of self or another person, or to seek to bring about justice on behalf of someone who cannot speak or act for himself. However, most conflict is simply a matter of a person not minding their own business. If you don't like something, leave the conversation or environment in which the conflict is taking place. Unless you—and other people involved—perceive that a conversation can be conducted in a rational, reasonable manner, don't start talking. There is little benefit in arguing or debating subjects without mutually agreeable conclusions or compromises. If you cannot compromise a position, walk away. Let your own life model the benefits of your opinions.

4. **Negative Words.** Watch what you say—at all times. I grew up in a world in which people routinely said, "Sticks and stones may hurt your bones but words can never hurt you." That, my friend, is a lie. Words can and

often do hurt. They can damage a person's self-value, dash a person's dreams, and destroy a person's reputation. The far better childhood saying to remember is this: "If you can't say something good about a person, don't say anything at all." Words spoken in an angry manner, or words that are aimed at hurting another person, nearly always produce a response of anger or vengeance, and once that cycle is started, it is very difficult to stop. If you have a choice between silence and rash statements, choose silence. And ... always refuse to become involved in idle gossip or speculation about another person's motives or character. You simply do not know all that you may *think* you know.

These four areas of emotional response to life: overspending and overextending, trying to control all situations and other people, engaging routinely in conflict, and speaking negatively are the MAJOR causes of emotional distress in the average person's life! And ALL of them are AVOIDABLE!

5. A Short Course on Insulin

A high blood pressure reading and a high BMI (body mass index) number often have one thing in common: too much INSULIN in the bloodstream. The hormone insulin signals the body to store fat, and it is the extra fat that is stored that increases BMI and clogs blood vessels, causing a construction of blood flow, and thus, a higher blood pressure reading.

The production of insulin is triggered by glucose (sugar) in the blood. Foods that break down quickly into sugar are the main culprits in causing a rapid and large amount of insulin to be released from the pancreas. Cells can only "use" the energy from glucose if the glucose is ushered into the cell by insulin. The main problem is that many of the foods we eat turn into sugar *too rapidly*. The Glycemic Index gets to the heart of this issue. Foods high on the Glycemic Index (larger numbers) are ones that break down very quickly and need more insulin. Those low on the Glycemic Index (smaller numbers) are ones that break down slowly and need less insulin.

Let me give you an example. A moderate sized potato has an index number of 84 (which is high), while a sweet potato the same size has an index number of 53 (medium). The sweet potato is the better choice.

The goal for every person should be to consume MOSTLY low to low/medium glycemic carbohydrates. Eat very few high Glycemic Index carbohydrates.

Overall, it is a good idea to limit carbohydrate consumption to "30 grams" per meal.

Stop all carbohydrate intake at least four hours before bedtime.

The goal of every person should be to trigger a *minimal* amount of insulin.

6. Don't Trust Decisions to Emotion

Don't trust your emotions when you make decisions. Your emotions were designed by God to trigger you into taking actions that result in greater justice and positive changes. If you rely on your emotions to give you direction in life, they will nearly always fail you. They are likely to lead you where you never wanted to go, make you say things you never wanted to say, make you do things you never wanted to do, and cause you to become someone you never wanted to become. Keep your emotions in check and subject them to the bright light of God's Word. Act on principles of truth, not "gut feelings."

This is not to say that intuition or discernment is not important. Rather, it is to say that *good* intuition will always be in line with God's truth, and good spiritual discernment will always be in keeping with what God's Word says is right and wrong.

7. Finding Stability in Chaos

For more than eleven years, I was a single father. I know that raising children is not a piece of cake, especially if you are doing it "on your own" without a mother in the home. I am grateful for the help my own mother gave me in the care of my children, and am even more grateful for the comfort I received from my relationship with God. The truth, however, is that on many days, I awoke either *certain* that I was going to have to face a difficult problem, or *certain* that there was a likelihood such a problem was going to rear its ugly head.

The big reality here is that life has problems. Nobody lives an "ideal" life, even if all the areas associated with wellness are in balance. You know some of MY story. Circumstances occur that rock our world—it might be anything from a natural catastrophe, or a major unavoidable accident, or a crime committed against you or a loved one. The negative results are very often material, physical, and emotional. Simultaneously.

So how do we find a center of "emotional stability" in the midst of what often seems like sheer chaos?

First, stay away from a "chemical" form of escape from your problems. Do NOT resort to the use of alcohol, drugs, or excess prescription medications to dull the pain you feel or to cloud the severity of a circumstance. In the end, that is only a means of ADDING to your problems, not solving them.

Second, if you are feeling the need to distract yourself from a negative circumstance, pick up a good book. I recently heard about a woman who seemed to find herself wide awake at about 2 AM night after night. She couldn't seem to get back to sleep, and she was afraid that if she took a sleeping pill she might not awaken early enough to get to work on time. So, she lay in her bed wide awake and resorted to what many people do in such a situation—she worried. She thought about all of the things that were wrong in her life and all of the things that might go wrong, and all of the negative consequences that *could* happen.

One night she said to herself, "Enough of this." She turned on the light, picked up an inspirational book, and began to read it. She decided that if she was going to be awake, at least she'd make good use of the time and be able to say to her sleepy self the next morning, "I did something productive." To her surprise, she felt positive and sleepy about thirty minutes later. She turned off the light, said, "Thank You, God" and went to sleep.

Two things were likely at work in this woman's life. The motivational book filled her mind with good ideas rather than worrisome ones. (It was fortunate, in my opinion, that she didn't pick up a book filled with immorality or violence.) She switched gears intellectually—from negative fears to positive hope. And then, she responded with gratitude to God. Again, this was a focus on what is RIGHT in life rather than what is problematic. A person cannot count their blessings and worry at the same time!

Third, reach out to positive people and immerse yourself in positive activities and situations. This can be as simple as picking up the phone or meeting a friend for lunch. It can mean engaging in a pleasurable hobby for a half hour a day. I know of a woman who was struggling to overcome an indebtedness that occurred in the wake of her husband's death. She began to be discouraged that she was too poor to go out with her friends to movies or to dinner ... at least temporarily. One day she looked across her living room and noticed the obvious: the baby grand piano in the corner of the room. She recalled the pleasure she once had felt in practicing the piano and hearing others play it. So she went to the piano, sat down, and began to play. She was a little surprised at how much of her piano-playing skill seemed to have disappeared, but that made her all the more committed to regaining her former skill. She emerged from her "poor period" (her terminology) not only playing the piano, but giving piano lessons to several of the neighborhood children—you guessed it, for enough money to enjoy a weekly outing with friends and make additional payments against her indebtedness.

It takes just as much effort to associate with a negative person as with a positive person. Choose to associate with positive people. Build friendships with those who share your beliefs and interests. Hang around people who are optimistic and with whom you can laugh.

Humor and laughter have a strong correlation with physical and emotional healing. If you fail in some way, learn to laugh at yourself, and then get up and try again. You truly CAN laugh your way all the way to wellness and wholeness!

You may want to revisit a hobby or activity you enjoyed as a child. I heard recently about an elderly man who had always been very physically active, but was now unable to do some of the chores he had once enjoyed (such as painting the house or pruning fruit trees). He didn't particularly enjoy reading, beyond the daily newspaper, or watching television late at night, so, he asked himself, "What did I like to do when I was a boy that I might be able to do now?" The answer was stamp collecting.

He bought a couple of reference books, a variety of stamps, a couple of albums, and began to build a new collection! It was more than an "activity" to do in the late-night hours. It was FUN. And it was an intellectual exercise as well. He read all of the information associated with each of the stamp issues and the birds, animals, people, or events being celebrated by postage stamp releases. He said later, "I had more to talk about with people than just the weather or latest sport scores. The result seemed to be that more people invited me to their homes for dinner parties, telling me I was "such a good conversationalist." I didn't dare tell them that I was learning from my stamp collection—I just smiled and said, 'Thank you.'"

Fourth, intentionally choose to cultivate a deeper spiritual life. For me, that meant—even in my busiest years—spending time in prayer and reading God's Word, and in attending church services with my children (where we heard inspirational messages and also were associating with the type of people I wanted my children both to know and to become like).

> A strong spirit usually leads a person to seek
> strength in every area of his or her life.

Fifth, maintain a healthful physical routine. No matter how bad circumstances around you may be, you CAN go for a brisk walk (take the baby in the stroller with you, or choose to exercise *with* your teenager) … you CAN cook dinner at home and invite other family members to work alongside you in chopping vegetables or grilling chicken breasts … you CAN watch wholesome videos with your children (that you can check out from the public library for free), or even read books aloud to each other (taking on some of the classic literature that you may have enjoyed as a child.

Maintain Hope and Faith. Are the five suggestions above a means of "denying" life's problems? No.

Are they an attempt to avoid of dealing with difficulties? No.

Are they ways of diminishing a problem? No.

Rather, they are means of finding a positive ray of hope and faith *in the midst of a difficult time.* They are ways of moving toward greater inner peace, rather than adding to the existing turmoil.

Always ask when you are feeling unsettled, discouraged, or down-hearted, "What is one thing I can do to feel BETTER physically, emotionally, or spiritually?" Then do that one thing.

There is never any advantage in doing something destructive or negative when you are already in a negative circumstance. You will only be adding to your own pain and taking the spiral staircase DOWN instead of up!

8. Develop "Uncommon" Courtesy

During a recent visit to the post office, I saw a woman holding several packages in her arms as she approached the entry doors. I moved quickly to open the door and hold it for her. She seemed shocked as she said, "Why, thank you, young man. People just don't do this anymore."

I was pleased she referred to me as a young man. But I had to agree with her when she pointed out that such a simple act of "common courtesy" may not be all that common these days.

Chivalry isn't dead unless you help kill it.

Here are ten very easy ways of showing courtesy to another person:

Open doors, especially for women and the elderly, or mothers who have young children in tow.

Return calls when you say you will.

Train yourself to say, "Yes, ma'am" and "yes, sir" ... and "no, ma'am" and "no, sir." Teach your children to do the same and role-model the behavior for them!

If you have spent an evening with a single person, call to make sure your guest gets home safely, especially if the weather is bad.

Offer a coat or blanket to a person who may be cold. If you like to keep the thermostat on the cool side in your home, have a stack of cozy blankets or lap robes handy to share with your guests.

Get the car if it is raining—don't ask your passengers to get wet along with you. Let them stand in a dry place while you do the running for the car.

Err on the side of being protective. That was the original motivation for men to walk on a sidewalk closest to traffic—not only to spare a lady friend from the splashes or possibility of danger from vehicles in the road, but also to take any hit of items that might be thrown from upstairs windows. Step in politely if you see that someone is being verbally mistreated or that a conflict is heating up. Try to be a source of peace.

Be predictable—it isn't being stodgy, it is being reliable.

Actively LISTEN when people are speaking. Don't just

pretend; truly show an interest. You'll likely learn something valuable in the process.

Don't seek to debate or argue if you disagree with a person. Listen to their opinion and if you are required to respond, you can always say, "You've given me something to think about."

Speak and Act with Respect. Voicing respect is also a form of courtesy. The more you VOICE respect for others, the more you will begin to respect yourself. Saying, "Yes, ma'am, no ma'am, yes sir, no sir, please, thank you, and I'm sorry" are expressions that convey RESPECT. I grew up with an understanding that doors were to be opened for ladies and men were to show courtesy in helping a woman with her coat and in seating a woman at a table. Men were expected to show RESPECT to women. Standing when an elder entered the room or came to your table in a restaurant was also a sign of RESPECT. I'm grateful for that upbringing. In showing respect to others, I developed greater respect for myself!

9. Overcoming a Commitment Phobia

A phobia is a deep fear, perhaps the most problematic kind of fear. Phobias tend to be extreme and irrational.

People often cite a fear of crowds, a fear of heights, or a fear of being stuck in an elevator. There is another type of phobia that gets less attention but is very damaging to a person's overall growth, development as a person, and well-being. It is the phobia related to making a "commitment."

172

The person with this type of phobia often holds to one or more of these beliefs:

- I deserve to be able to live without making any commitments.

- I shouldn't have to make a commitment to work hard—life should be easier, not harder.

- There's got to be a shortcut to success that I'm overlooking (or a shortcut to a better relationship, a better job, a better life).

- God will supply all I need without my doing anything.

- People owe me—I shouldn't have to make any commitments to others; they should be making commitments to *me*.

- Commitment has nothing to do with my feelings or another person's ability to trust me.

- I am entitled to this because … (and you fill in the blanks).

These statements are wrong, wrong, wrong, and oh so wrong.

The truth of life, however, is that nobody *owes* you anything. For that matter, God your Creator does not *owe* you anything. Nothing that we ever attain or achieve related to tasks or relationships comes without a genuine heart commitment to setting and pursuing a goal, and being consistent in our efforts until we achieve a goal.

That's true for a good friendship, a good marriage, a good

relationship with one's children, the development of a good career, the pursuit of health and wellness, the attainment of a degree or skill or the development of a talent to a level of excellence. Neither do effective ministries or a stable psychological or emotional state come without a commitment to their pursuit.

Ask yourself these questions:

- Are you afraid of a commitment, perhaps because you fear failure?

- Do you have a negative response to goals because you have set them in the past and didn't achieve them?

- Do you resent those who set goals and achieve them?

- Do you feel an aversion to all forms of *challenges*, even ones you set for yourself?

- Do you want more out of your life, or are you satisfied with your current state of being?

These are questions only you can answer.

Some of the ways to move beyond commitment phobia are:

1. Give yourself permission to fail. Nobody is perfect and from time to time, you *will* fail. It is a fact of life. The fact also exists that *you*, and only you, determine the full extent to which you will learn from those failures and the number of times you will choose to pick yourself up after a fall and try again.

2. Learn to forgive yourself. Every person has need in his or her life to forgive others, to receive forgiveness from

others, and especially to forgive one's own self. Develop the practice of forgiving freely and generously.

3. Focus on something in your life that you want to achieve to the point that you are *willing* to put out some extra effort to attain it.

4. Discover your own innate talents and gifts—the abilities you seem to have had since birth. Your Creator has built into you an ability to do one or more things (skills) and succeed in development of them to a point of excellence. Focus on what you have been "gifted" to do and develop those talents. They are the areas in which you will find the greatest pleasure and satisfaction, and also be the areas in which you will be best able to bless the lives of others.

5. The mark of a champion is in getting up off the mat even when the referee is about to count you out.

Don't let feelings of fear of ANY type keep you from *anything* that you know is for your benefit—now or in the future, and especially those things that are for your eternal benefit!

---

10. Don't Hurt Your Children

Most parents have a deep desire to help their children, not hurt them. Child abuse is a horror to a child and a blight on our society. The vast majority of parents would never want to think of themselves as abusive or hurtful in any way. The sad truth, however, is that many parents hurt their children without even realizing they are doing so. Here are six of the main ways I have seen parents do the "wrong things" for their child or children:

1. They give their children candy and other forms of sweets (such as sugar-loaded beverages) in order to placate their demands. Children often ask their parents for all sorts of things that aren't good for them, and it is a part of good parenting to say, "No" and then provide a nutritious alternative or to insist the child wait for their next mealtime. Candy not only rots teeth but creates an addictive cycle of sugar highs and lows that can greatly damage a child's health, and even lead to childhood obesity or early-onset diabetes. Candy should especially be avoided as a "reward"—it is actually a punishment in disguise.

2. They resort to the nearest fast-food drive-through rather than take the time and make the effort to prepare a nutritious meal at home. Most parents need to take better control of their own schedules and plan for family dinner times. The "food" will likely be more tasty, more nutritious, and the conversation around the dinner table can also be a form of emotional, intellectual, and spiritual "feeding."

3. They allow a child to order what the child wants from

a menu, in whatever form of restaurant they find themselves. Take responsibility for selecting what your child will eat. If you want to give your child a choice or a lesson in decision-making, narrow their options to one or two alternatives.

4. They cook to placate a child's demands rather than insist that a child eat what has been prepared. At the very minimum, a child should be required to try a new food before deciding it isn't to the child's liking. Parents, of course, can help their cause by learning to prepare food in appetizing ways, and to show their own enjoyment for a particular food. Don't insist that your child eat what you won't eat. Be aware that texture is just as important to a child as "taste." Your child may not like things that are "runny," "lumpy," "stringy," or "slimy." Most adults don't like these textures either. You CAN fix foods that are good in texture without tossing out a food as being undesirable.

5. They plug their children into various electronics rather than encourage them to engage in physical activity or creative play. They are doing a disservice to the child's health, they are curtailing their emotional ability to play with others, and they are short-circuiting their intellectual ability to make up their own plotlines and create their own props and sets.

6. They smile at their child's "chubbiness." In many cases,

parents ignore their child's obesity because the parent is also obese. Excess weight is a detriment to flexibility, motivation, endurance, and overall energy levels—in both children and adults. To ignore the health risks of obesity is often to set up a child for a lifetime of struggling to lose weight or maintain healthy weight.

You can kill anything with neglect, including a child.

---

11. Seek to Be a Person of Integrity

Do you have a good definition for the word "integrity"? If not, here's the dictionary definition:

- A firm adherence to a code of values.

- Incorruptibility—an unimpaired condition of soundness.

- The quality or state of being complete and undivided—especially without division between belief and behavior.

Integrity is a word that speaks to all that we hold as good character, morality, and upright living.

There are several keys to living a life of integrity. I offer you these as my top six suggestions:

1. Choose your words carefully. Say what you believe, and only what you believe. Pause before you speak. Think about an answer before you give one. Let your yes be yes, and your no be no.

2. Respect the time of others. Show up for appointments on time. Value the "gift of time" that others give you.

3. Pay your bills. Give others who have rendered service or provided goods for you what they are rightfully owed.

4. Be courteous. There's never a good excuse for bad manners. Say please and thank you. Display respect in the way you treat others.

5. Own up to your own failures and take responsibility for mistakes you make.

6. Apologize readily. Forgive freely and ask for forgiveness if you are the offending party. And once you have apologized and been forgiven, or once another person has apologized and you have forgiven, let the matter go. Don't bring it up again ... ever.

Integrity is built one bit of behavior at a time. It is difficult to maintain and easy to destroy. Guard your integrity. It will become your reputation, and ultimately, your legacy.

Having a failure does not mean you ARE a failure. Making a mistake does not mean your life is a mistake. Sinning doesn't ever mean that you are beyond God's forgiveness.

---

12. How to Live a Relatively Debt-Free Life

One of the best rules for life that I know is this:

Live in Agreement with Your Assets

If you do this, you will have the money to pay your bills and to live a relatively debt-free life. I say "relatively debt free" because most people will never be able to live totally debt free. As one person put it, "There's always dirty laundry to wash and there's always the utility bill to be paid!"

Most people have long-term financial commitments, such as a home mortgage.

"Debt free" is defined by a number of financial advisors as having the ability to pay your normal monthly expenses, including a mortgage payment, without increasing your overall financial liability or debt load.

To live a relatively debt-free life you need to budget the money that you earn and choose to live by that budget, not extending your expenses beyond your income. In addition, you will be wise to:

- Work hard and stay committed to your job. It is generally easier to keep a job than to get a new job. And, it is generally easier to find a better job if you already have a job.

- Give a percentage of your income to charity. To some people, this makes no sense. In the end, however, giving to those who are *less* fortunate places a greater focus on what a giver has, and in many cases, motivates a giver to be wiser and less reckless in managing his or her resources.

- Set aside a percentage of what is earned for long-range savings, to help through future emergencies or retirement years.

- "Pay" yourself a small amount for enjoyment activities, such as entertainment or travel. Then, go for that pleasurable experience when you can pay cash. By paying yourself in advance, you will avoid putting "pleasure" on a credit card and paying far more in the end for the same trip or activity.

13. Taking a Salad to Work

I truly believe that one of the best investments a person can make is a small personal-sized refrigerator that can be discreetly set into a person's office. Use it for storing protein drinks, water bottles, several pieces of fresh fruit, and bring-your-lunch meals.

Meals you bring from home are often better tasting and less expensive than ones purchased at a restaurant—not always, but often.

Eating a made-at-home salad with 5–6 ounces of lean protein (such as water-packed albacore or a chicken breast) will generally cost between $8 and $12, including tip, in a restaurant. The bring-from-home price can be as little as $4 to $5.

I am not recommending that you eat at your desk or that

you try to double task by eating and doing work at the same time. Rather, I recommend you take your salad to a location outside your office, preferably one with a view you enjoy and perhaps even outside your office building to a nearby park. Or, if you do stay in your office, use the extra time after you eat to read something non-work related, tackle a crossword or Sudoku puzzle, or even put your head down on your desk and take a ten-minute nap.

The Cost of "Wellness" Food. While thinking about the cost of a "bring-from-home salad," we may as well address the issue of the COST of purchasing high-quality foods that contribute to good health.

I readily admit that making the switch to whole and real foods MAY increase your grocery budget by twenty to thirty percent INITIALLY. This is owing to the fact that many people have to empty most of their pantries when they make a commitment to eating real food without excessive processing and un-pronounceable chemical additives. Over time, however, eating whole and real foods generally results in people eating LESS food as a whole (and feeling more satisfied at the same time), and over time, the cost is going to be the same, perhaps even less.

The Temptation Factor. A little discussed factor related to bring-from-home meals is the "temptation factor." When a person goes to a restaurant, he or she is often subjected to peer pressure that results in ordering foods, including dessert, the person might not otherwise order. And there is nearly always a "temptation factor" related to salad dressings, croutons, pasta salads on the salad bar, and various meat and vegetable items swimming in delectable sauces.

Do You Need a Gym Membership?

Maybe not. And I rarely recommend that a gym membership be an initial part of, or a prerequisite for, a Wellness Plan. I consider my local gym to be my personal "exercise room." It beats the cost of adding one to my house.

The truth is ... a gym membership is only worth the cost if you will go to the gym regularly and avail yourself of the services offered by the staff there, including personal trainers. If you only want to ride a stationary bike, you can buy a bike and save yourself a lot of money over the course of a couple years.

Many good exercise programs can be done at home, or in your neighborhood. It often helps to have a DVD to motivate you into doing a variety of exercises, perhaps with the advantage of "how-to" tips and a little music in the background. Good strength-training exercises can be done using the walls, chairs, and countertops of your own living room and kitchen! Climbing the stairs in your home, or walking in a nearby shopping mall, are good forms of exercise that most people can readily do.

Remember always that the best exercise for you is ... *the one you will do!*

[And yes, I do have exercise DVDs. Check out my website if you are interested at www.live4E.com]

15. Good Risk Management

I once had a client who worked in the insurance industry in the area of "risk management." He told me that he thought the Wellness Plan I was teaching was one of the best "risk management programs" he had ever encountered. I agreed!

The facts confirm:

- If a person eats sensibly and correctly, he lowers the "probability" of acquiring diabetes before the age of seventy.

- If a person exercises regularly, she decreases her risk of having cardiovascular disease.

- If a person maintains proper posture while standing and sitting, he lowers the "probability" of back troubles.

- If a person gets proper rest, she decreases her "risk" of becoming fatigued.

- If a person stops texting or using the phone while driving, he decreases the "odds" of causing a traffic collision.

- If a person chooses to be reckless in the area of nutrition, opting for a sedentary life and not getting enough rest or sufficient exercise, that person increases the "probability" of premature death or a highly impaired quality of life.

Perhaps we will eventually get to the place where we award people for good health management, and reduce our national health-care expenditures as a byproduct. With certainty, those who take a proactive approach to good healthcare are *likely* to enjoy a better quality of life for more years than those who don't. The stats are in their favor!

16. The Need for Wellness in the Religious World

"Wellness" is a concept that I believe firmly should become a common topic of conversation and teaching, as well as practical programs related to conduct and outreach, in every church or synagogue in our nation. It is at the very heart of what God's Word describes as "being made *whole*."

If anybody needs wellness, it is those in church leadership. In a widely published research study, the results below were cited:

- 13% of active pastors are divorced

- Discouragement runs high among the clergy. Almost a quarter of pastors are fired or pressured to resign at least once in their career.

- About a quarter of pastors' wives resent their husband's work schedule and about a quarter feel they have nowhere to turn if they have a family or personal crisis, or marriage conflict.

- About a third of all pastors feel burned out after their first five years of ministry.

- About a third of pastors believe that being in ministry is a "hazard" to their family members emotionally, psychologically, or spiritually.

- 45% of pastors report feeling depression and about half say they feel "unable" to meet all the needs of the job they face.

- 70% say they have no close friends and 75% report feeling severe stress much of the time (including feeling anguish, worry, bewilderment, anger, depression, fear, and alienation).

- About 90% feel unqualified or poorly prepared for ministry.

- 94% feel pressure to have a perfect family.

Pastors, along with doctors and lawyers, have the most problems of any career group when it comes to drug abuse, alcoholism, and suicide.

If you are a pastor, priest, or rabbi, the best thing you can do for yourself and your followers is to develop a personal WELLNESS plan.

And … the second-best thing you can do is to teach and share this WELLNESS plan with those who are part of your spiritual flock.

8

Ongoing Steps — Phase 3

I WANT TO MAKE one thing very clear as you prepare to move into Phase 3 of your wellness program—this is not the final lap of a race. It is not entering the stadium as the final phase of a marathon. There is no END to Phase 3, no finish line, no coronation ceremony. Phase 3 is the way you should WANT to live for the rest of your life!

As I previously advised before you began Phase 2, I recommend that a person stay with the goals and activities associated with Phase 2 of their Wellness Plan for a full month before setting out to tackle the behaviors identified in Phase 3. This gives time for previously undetected problems to surface, and for the person to renew their commitment to pursuing an additional set of goals and healthful behaviors.

All of the activities in Phase 3 are built upon those in Phases 1 and 2. In some cases, more time or greater quantity is

The activities in Phase 3 are built upon those in Phase 2. Continue to do those things you began in earlier phases.

ONGOING STEPS —

PHYSICAL

- Eliminate processed foods
- Eliminate gluten and MSG
- Make a commitment to changing your nutritional plan to focus on natural, raw, and whole foods
- Monitor your protein choices and add a high-quality protein drink to your daily eating plan
- Add stretching and flexibility exercises to your exercise plan
- Give up all toxins (including tobacco)
- Pay attention to your posture (sitting, standing, walking)
- Add supplements if you need them

EMOTIONAL

- Make a TIME budget (monthly)
- Declutter your living space, car, and office
- Go on a regular vacation with your family (at least 2–3 days every 2 months)
- Drop unhealthy relationships
- Embark on an active plan to pre-habilitate your life
- Go on an outing with a select group of friends at least once every three months

Set Goals + Consolidate and Balance + Reset Goals +

recommended, but previous behaviors are never entirely set aside. Don't lose sight of that principle!

If a suggestion on these pages involves more time or a greater quantity, make that adjustment.

PHASE 3

INTELLECTUAL

- Explore the full spectrum of your personal talents or "giftedness"

- Do something at least once every three months that is a "learning" event (conference, retreat, short course, special lecture)

- Expand your circle of mentors and wise counselors

SPIRITUAL

- Begin to help others in regular volunteer service

Get Counseling if you need it + Keep a Personal Journal

Notes about the PHYSICAL Dimension of Phase 3

1. Eliminate all processed foods.

2. Eliminate gluten and MSG.

Another way of saying "processed" is pre-packaged. Anything that comes in a box (including frozen food containers) has been processed in ways that diminish the nutritional value of the ingredients.

Not all processed foods have gluten or MSG, but many do. Wherever you find MSG, avoid it. (Some Oriental restaurants still use MSG in their dishes.) At least one neurosurgeon (a brain surgeon) calls MSG an "exito-toxin." It not only is toxic to the brain but it excites various neurotransmitters in the brain to go rogue. Not good.

Gluten. We hear a lot about gluten today. Gluten is not natural to food. It is often added to promote strength or stickiness to food, especially to wheat and other grains, and thus, to help with the rising of dough and to give breads more "chewiness." There are many foods manufactured with added gluten, including:
- Soups
- Croutons and bread crumbs
- Some candies
- Fried foods
- Imitation fish
- Some lunch meats, including hot dogs

- Seasoned chips
- Salad dressings
- Soy sauce
- Seasoned rice

The side effects in the body are not pleasant. They can include:

- Abdominal bloating
- Abnormal stools
- Calcium metabolism disturbance
- Constipation
- Flatulence (gas)
- Intestinal malabsorption
- Muscle wasting
- Poor appetite
- Irritability
- Impaired growth
- Iron deficiency anemia
- Poor muscle tone

Celiac disease may result from gluten intolerance. Many immune-system diseases can also be impacted by gluten.

3. COMMIT to natural, raw, and whole foods.

We've advocated natural, raw, and whole throughout this book but now is your time to COMMIT to eating *only* natural, raw, and whole foods AS MUCH AS POSSIBLE.

One of my clients said recently, "Dr. Mark, this is actually the easiest thing you've asked me to do. I simply changed where

I shop for groceries. I go to a place that only sells natural, raw, and whole foods!" Fortunately, more and more of those grocery outlets are available.

4. Have a protein drink for breakfast.

I am a great fan of protein drinks.

I encourage people to make a powdered protein drink with 20–25 grams of high quality whey protein mixed with 12–14 ounces of unsweetened almond or coconut milk. This highly dense drink will give you a good start to the day and help you maintain energy and regulate blood sugar well into the late afternoon. Those who routinely have a protein drink like this in the morning consume fewer calories during the remainder of the day than those who start out with no breakfast or a meal that has sugary foods.

5. Add mobility and flexibility exercises.

Mobility is an important way to maintain your flexibility and also to avoid injuries while doing other types of exercise. We must learn to move in correct patterns of motion. Mobility allows flexibility. Flexibility is the degree to which tendons and ligaments stretch.

The time to stretch is AFTER your muscles are "warmed up" to a degree. Don't stretch cold muscles—it is like stretching a rubber band that has been in a freezer. ("Breaking" is a lot more common.) Walk for five to ten minutes and THEN stretch, perhaps before you shift to a race-walk speed, jogging, or running.

Always stretch s-l-o-w-l-y until you get to the full extension of your stretch. Stretching not only helps your muscles, it helps your circulation.

The best thing to do when you awaken in the morning is to do some slow stretches before you get out of bed (and while your body is still warm from being under the covers). Take a look at the way dogs and cats "awaken" after a nap. They nearly always s-t-r-e-t-c-h. Human babies tend to do the same thing. Learn from them!

6. Give up all toxins.

Don't breathe in chemicals of any kind if you can possibly avoid them.

Stop all tobacco use, drug use, use of heavy-duty prescription drugs (ask your doctor to help you wean off them), and any other chemical on which you suspect you may have become addicted. Get free!

7. Add supplements.

The *majority* of people can benefit from at least some vitamin and mineral supplementation in their daily eating plan. That's because our soil isn't what it used to be and many minerals have been leached away. Furthermore, most food processing seriously damages or destroys vitamins and minerals.

People often ask me what I consider to be the most important supplements for most people. Here are my top ten suggestions:

1. **Protein powder.** Take about 30–40 grams in the form of a protein drink. Add "greens" to enhance nutritional value. Blend thoroughly! Not all protein powders are created equal. Some options include whey, pea, beef, hemp, and others (food allergies and sensitivities are factors along with preferred food plans – vegetarian).

2. **Fish oil.** An excellent supplement to fight inflammation and generate heart and brain health. Choose a triglyceride-bound source that is high in Omega 3s (EPA and DHA). I like a product that has lipase—a digestive enzyme suspended in a gel cap form. I recommend 2–4 grams for women and 4–6 grams for men. The fish oil quality is vital to absorption.

3. **CoQ10.** Select the ubiquinone form. CoQ10 is critical to energy production of the mitochondria (the cell's powerhouse of energy production) and for the nervous system. Further, CoQ10 gets depleted with age, exercise, and statin drug use. A daily dose of 50–100 mg is recommended. Some individuals may require higher doses as recommended by their primary physician.

4. **Vitamin D3 (cholecalciferol).** Most people are deficient in this. I recommend 1000–5000 IU for maintenance of this vitamin in the body as a base. If a person is deficient, this may require up to 10,000 IU until an adequate level is reached. Vitamin D helps with sleep, acts as a hormonal aid, moderates immune function, helps with

bone health, and assists with overall energy and nervous system health. It may also decrease musculoskeletal pain.

5. **Vitamin C.** Extremely important for immune health, connection tissue, and skin integrity. I like a powder form so that I can add it to my protein shakes. I recommend 1–2 grams a day.

6. **Magnesium-Calcium.** These two work together in the body to help with cellular energy and bone health. Magnesium is actually required by the body for more than 350 metabolic reactions! Magnesium deficiency is very common.

7. **Glutamine.** This is the #1 amino acid used by cells in the intestine. It is very important for gastrointestinal health and digestion. It also aids in the regeneration of muscle tissue after exercise.

8. **Probiotics.** These aid digestion and are an important source of Vitamin K2 (which helps with the absorption of Vitamin D in generating bone health). They are also very important for the immune system of the gut and ecology.

9. **Basic multivitamin.** Multifunctional and broad-based, with both vitamins and minerals.

10. **Full-spectrum antioxidant.** Important for the prevention of free-radical damage and for overcoming toxic waste in the body.

Notes about the EMOTIONAL Dimension of Phase 3

Make a time budget.

This is similar to a financial budget only allocating hours and minutes rather than dollars and cents.

Every person gets 1440 minutes a day. No more. There could be less (and likely will be on the day you die) but there are no more.

Every person decides how to manage their minutes—at least the majority of them. We have the privilege in our society of choosing some activities over others, and with different time priorities allotted to our choices.

Just as we cannot spend more than we make—at least not for long—so we cannot make bad time choices without negative consequences.

There truly is a major advantage to "paying yourself first." We know that in building a good retirement plan or investment portfolio. We know that when it comes to putting on an oxygen mask before helping the person next to us put on his. In terms of time management, the person who chooses to invest in things that have long-range value, and especially those things that promise eternal rewards, is going to be much happier with his life in the future than the person who has no regard for today's time choices.

Time management is a challenge for every person. How are you going to make the most of the time *you* are given in a day?

Time Management Tips. Here are six suggestions for better management of your time:

1. Plan your day the night before. Make a check list of things you intend to do the next day. Set your alarm clock for fifteen minutes earlier than you THINK you need to.

2. Set two alarms in the morning. If one doesn't do the trick, the other might! Set the second alarm far enough away from your bed that you have to get up in order to turn it off.

3. Write down your to-do list. Don't try to hold it in memory. (You *will* forget something important … at some time … and generally when it is most embarrassing.)

4. Prioritize your to-do list. Don't just brain-dump all you'd *like* to do. Put things in priority order. Then choose to do the first thing first, and so on through the list. Put the least-important things to do at the bottom of your list, and in that position, if you don't get to these things, you have left the "least important" things undone, not the MOST important things undone.

5. Put out your clothes for the following day, including socks and shoes. You'll likely only save a few minutes here and there, but they all add up over a week!

6. End your day with a calming period of silence. This allows your mind to rest even as you are preparing for your

body to sleep. Don't rehearse what you didn't get done or what you intend to do the next day. Focus, instead, on the good moments of the day that is behind you.

1. Declutter your life.

Clutter confuses the average person—it scatters focus.

Clutter takes time—time finding things, time moving things to get to other things, time preparing a space for other people.

Clutter often distracts a person from a task that is under a "deadline."

Clutter annoys those with whom you may work or live.

Get things organized and keep them that way. You'll be sending a message to your brain that your Wellness Plan is going to be a prime way that you "declutter" your body, mind, emotions, and spirit. Make way for the end of confusion and the establishment of clarity and order!

2. Take vacations with your family.

There is nothing noble about refusing to have leisure time in your life. Every person needs time "off" and ideally, time "away" from the pressures of a job.

Time apart from the grind of a job's responsibilities can help a person rejuvenate physically and emotionally, and also reconnect with loved ones (family members or close friends). Time apart from a job's chores can also help a person gain a greater perspective on life, reprioritize goals, and dream new dreams.

Your family especially needs to connect with you apart from your work life. I highly recommend 2–3 days spent with your family every 2 months. That can be a long weekend, or mid-week days during a school break, or any other period that fits into *your* family schedule. Go someplace to have FUN. Unplug all electronic devices and talk to one another. Create opportunities for laughter and adventure.

3. Go on outings with selected friends.

Friendships also can benefit from "retreat" times in which there is no agenda *other* than friendship. Spend time in casual but prolonged conversation. Again, make room for lots of laughter!

Marriages, parent-child relationships, and friendships all need heavy doses of nurturing and time in order to grow and flourish.

4. Drop unhealthy relationships.

We all know the line in one of Robert Frost's poems: "Good fences make good neighbors." It's true! And when it comes to relationships of all kinds—from casual friendships to the intimacy of marriage—good relationships need good boundaries.

Perhaps the foremost word to keep in mind when it comes to setting boundaries is this:

No.

No is a complete sentence. It is vital that you learn to use this word any time you are being asked to do something that is against your own code of ethics, your deepest beliefs, or that is something that has little chance of succeeding or being fulfilling to you.

If you sense that somebody is trying to get you to do their work or to get something for nothing ... run, don't walk, in separating yourself from that person's influence.

Keep in mind that manipulative people are often fairly subtle. They use a variety of tactics—from a "guilt trip" to a "pleading look" to "teary eyes" to "a forlorn sounding voice" to a fictitious but real-sounding scenario—to get you to do what they want, which is nearly always 90 percent for their benefit.

There are some people who can suck the very life out of you if you let them. You KNOW who they are! Learn to say NO to their requests, and if it makes you feel better, you can say, "No, thank you," or, "No, I don't believe that is the right thing for me to do," or even, "No, I don't think that is the choice I should make right now." But be firm and don't leave room for being talked into something you truly do not value, do not want, or do not seek.

In saying "no" to manipulative people, you are not only doing yourself a favor, but you are generally freeing yourself up to say "yes" to people you truly can help, do want to spend time with, and with whom you can develop an "interdependence" marked by mutual help, respect, and commitment.

The word "no" may seem harsh or negative to you, but keep in mind that the person who says "no" is very likely opening himself or herself to saying "yes" to something positive, and far more nourishing and satisfying than the present reality. Saying "no" may be the necessary prerequisite for saying "yes."

5. PREhabilitate your life.

Most people are familiar with rehabilitation. It's what a person does AFTER an accident, serious surgery, or in pursuit of recovery from an addiction.

PREhabilitation is what a person might do BEFORE an emergency arises in their life to be in the best possible position for a speedy, efficient, and full recovery if an emergency arises.

Pre-habilitation is "the management style of incorporating proactive and preventative measures or actions designed to PREVENT mistakes, delays, deficiencies, and the development of an unwanted business culture BEFORE they occur."

If you could prevent bankruptcy, wouldn't you?

If you could avoid the pain of a divorce, wouldn't you?

If you could escape having a serious heart attack or debilitating stroke, wouldn't you?

Most people will respond with a resounding YES.

Much of pre-habilitation lies in the realm of EMOTIONAL WELLNESS.

Pre-habilitate Your Finances. Debt avoidance and thus, bankruptcy avoidance, begins with the formation of a budget. If you don't know how to make one, ask a financial advisor or a close personal friend who manages money well to help you make a budget. There are also a number of self-help manuals and books that can help with this process.

Most people need *some* help managing money at various times in their life. Generally speaking, people need help in planning their estates, and increasingly it seems, help in doing their taxes. Many people need help in choosing the right investments to make with their "savings" and other discretionary income or windfalls (perhaps from an inheritance).

Don't be afraid to ask for help, and don't begrudge paying a fair fee for these services. A good financial advisor should end up helping you MAKE or KEEP money, not take all your money.

Pre-habilitate Your Relationships. Every good relationship takes time and effort—no matter how good that relationship may be at the outset or how good it may be presently. Even a *very good* relationship needs time and effort to maintain its goodness moving forward!

Seek to develop two to five CLOSE friends with whom you can share deeply your feelings, thoughts, and goals. Choose people who will keep your confidences and affirm you without agreeing to every whim you voice.

Periodically spend a concentrated time apart from the world with these friends, and if you are married, a concentrated time apart from the world with your spouse. (These times are not the *same* times!)

Give yourself the opportunity to relax together, dream your respective futures, and enter into deeper-than-usual conversations. You may want time set aside for prayer, or for doing together a relaxing activity you enjoy.

Friends and marriages that "play" together are nearly always stronger and more vibrant.

Find something that you and your spouse enjoy doing together that can become a focal for an ongoing "dating" relationship between the two of you. I know of one couple who belonged to a square-dance club for thirty years, going to various barn dances once every week or two. Yes, frilly dresses and string ties included. They loved dancing together! Another couple I know has recently joined a gourmet cooking club. They are looking for new ways to make "whole real foods" even more tasty. Good for them. They take genuine delight in cooking for and with each other!

Find things that renew and enhance real *friendship*.

Pre-habilitate Your Health. Virtually all of the PHYSICAL portions of the Wellness Plan are aimed at pre-habilitation. There are three keys to this that are important to remember:

- Schedule time for your fitness just as you would schedule a business appointment.

- Have regular physical checkups with a physician or trainer, and regular times to take your "vital" signs (weight, cholesterol, blood pressure).

- Make friends who are also pursuing a wellness plan. Share tips with them, including healthful recipes and strategies for maintaining good practices in difficult circumstances.

Pre-habilitate Your Business. If you are leading a wellness plan in your company, suggest that pre-habilitation be considered a "management" style—it is always better to anticipate a failure and plan for recovery from it than to find yourself in a crisis moment. Just as "crisis management" is considered a bad way to manage, pre-habilitation management might be considered the best way to manage.

Pre-habilitation does not cause a person to deny that bad outcomes may arise from even the best of efforts. Rather, it says, "Let's have a strategy for dealing with setbacks, downturns, or unforeseen circumstances."

One man told a friend of mine that he calls this a "hurricane plan." This man had lived in the southeastern part of the United States in a coastal community. He pointed out to me that virtually all of the towns and cities had predesignated evacuation routes in case of a hurricane—signs already posted, a map readily available to any person desiring one.

He also noted that since the signs had gone up and the maps had been distributed about ten years ago, his particular city had not experienced a hurricane. "But," he quickly added, "we all feel ready should one come our way. It gives us a little more peace as we go about our daily lives and enjoy our rounds of golf."

This same thing is true for having a transition plan, or in the case of personal estate planning, a will or living trust. Once these plans or documents are in place, there's generally a greater sense of peace that a person will know what to do if, or when, a negative circumstance arises. Even if the plan needs to be adjusted after a crisis hits, there's a good result that usually comes from a group of people *planning together* to solve a potential problem or meet a possible need. Communication patterns and relationships are established that are generally very helpful down the road, with or without a crisis.

Pre-habilitate Your Family's Safety. I have a friend who grew up in California and still has many relatives and friends in that state. She told me recently about the five-gallon-bucket plan that is in place in most schools and in many families throughout southern California. Every family has certain emergency items set aside in a five-gallon bucket that can be picked up quickly and easily should evacuation from a home be required (in face of a forest fire, flooding situation, or earthquake). Every person in the family or school knows where the bucket(s) are located. Nobody uses the items in the bucket along the way, even if duplicate items need to be purchased for normal everyday use.

Those who live in areas prone to tornadoes know the advantage of having adequate storm shelters. Those who live near rivers or along coastal areas know the advantage of building homes with materials and foundation supports that can withstand storm surges and strong winds. "Be prepared" is a good motto for all good citizens, not just good scouts.

In developing a pre-habilitation plan for your family, make sure that you have a plan for how to communicate with one another if all cell phones become inoperable, electricity goes out, and key roads may be blocked. Where will you go? How will you get to the meeting place you designate? Who will you turn to for information or assistance?

There's yet another aspect of pre-habilitation for a family and that is pre-habilitation related to behavior and communication.

The Pre-habilitative Power of Communication. Choose to have "talk and listen" sessions with your children. You may call these family meetings. Take time to discuss issues that are facing you as a family—such as how to assign chores for the coming month, where you might want to consider going on vacation, how you are going to schedule after-school activities and transportation to and from then. Use this time to voice concerns that may be arising in the family. This is a time to underscore certain family rules, clarify opinions, express gratitude, and discuss relationship problems.

Give each person a slot for "talking" during the meeting. Insist on polite listening and no interruptions while a person is talking. If you can't resolve a difference of opinions during one meeting, set a time to meet again, perhaps on a focused topic (such as dealing with WHO is going to be responsible for feeding the pets and what the consequences will be for not doing so).

Have *individual* communication times for dealing with one particular child's bad behavior or negative school reports as well as time for directed praise.

As much as possible, eat together as a family in the evenings. Turn off the television, sit at the family dining table together, and enjoy sharing the highlights of your respective days—including the problems, struggles, issues with friends and teachers, and challenges that lie ahead (such as that ten-page term paper due in six weeks). Make sure every person feels free to talk and refuse to allow interruptions or "talking over each other." A table can be set, food eaten, and the table cleared within thirty minutes. It will be a time worth scheduling and maintaining as a family tradition!

Pre-habilitating a Marriage. I have seen serious disasters result from people who married without becoming well acquainted. I recommend that a person date another for at least 1–2 years before entering marriage, and during this time, to remain celibate and apart from each other sexually. This flies in the face of virtually all that the media and movie world have to say. However, a good relationship for a *lifetime* is not limited to sexual attraction or even to having mutual dreams. It is related in genuine compatibility of values and beliefs, a genuine enjoyment of each other's personality, and a genuine ability to live a life that has mutually appreciated activities and traditions. It takes time to make these discoveries about another person, and to see another person in times of both failure and success, tragedy and joy, and crises and pleasure.

Don't overlook or underplay the importance of good pre-marital counseling with a pastor or licensed family counselor. You will likely face questions in such sessions that you never thought to ask or felt too embarrassed to ask.

Pre-habilitating Your Work Environment. A high percentage of "working relationships" can be pre-habilitated by the setting of boundaries —this is true for both career-related work environments and various volunteer or committee-related tasks.

Healthy boundaries should be marked and defined early on. If boundaries become muddled or unclear, it is much more difficult to RESET boundaries than to set them properly at the outset.

This goes beyond "job descriptions," although they are a part of setting boundaries. In boundary-setting, communication lines as well as topics can be *clearly* delineated, in addition to a general protocol for how to relate to others in general ways within the company, clinic, committee, and so forth.

It is generally best NOT to devote work or task-related time to the sharing of personal information or problems. If a co-worker wants to talk about personal issues, be polite but listen only with limits. It is not your job to be the person's counselor (unless that IS your job as a licensed professional counselor). Suggest, if it is appropriate, that the person avail himself or herself of professional counseling opportunities, some of which may be currently in place at your company or organization.

I heard not long ago about a church that nearly dissolved because boundaries had not been set clearly between the incoming pastor and the church board. In the several months that the church had been without a full-time pastor, the board had assumed all responsibilities related to the revision of the church's doctrinal positions and protocol with regional and national leaders, clearly establishing the board as being in charge of the pastor rather than the pastor being the leader of the board. This was not at all the position of the denomination as a whole. (While that ordering of responsibility and authority may be present in *some* denominations, it was not the policy in this denomination.) The board leaders refused to back down, bishops got involved, and the newly hired pastor came very close to walking away. Boundaries needed to be reset, and reset quickly, for this church to survive.

In a similar but different setting, I also heard recently about a church body that had fallen into the habit of referring to every person by their first name, including the church leaders. Everything seemed very "chummy," as one member of the church said. But with that degree of familiarity came a degree of assuming genuine friendship. A leader can be a personal friend with only so many people, and in a church setting, those friendships are not likely to be with church members. Furthermore, the first-name practice seemed to erode a sense of respect for the spiritual authority and responsibilities of the church leader. It almost became as if "everyone" was a pastor or leader in the church. It didn't work. Boundaries needed to be reset, and it was not an easy transition.

These issues of familiarity and policy control are not unique to churches, of course. The same can apply to virtually all professions and groups of people organized to engage in ongoing relationships and task-completion. There is always going to be a hierarchy—formal or informal—if decision-making is involved.

It is a good personal policy to choose to be friendly with all in your work environment, not just a few. The clique group that is "in" today may be "out" tomorrow!

There are several basic workplace rules that apply to all good task-completion environments:

- Arrive on time, and being a little early won't hurt. Employers or leaders can usually accommodate the occasional emergency that causes a person on the "team" to be late, but habitual tardiness is nearly always resented and can impact a person's position within the organization.

- Work the full time you have been hired to work. If that's eight hours a day, work the full eight hours. Make sure you keep your break and lunch times within the established time slots.

- Be courteous and polite to every person in the organization, as well as to all customers or vendors who may come in and out of your work environment.

- Avoid idle chatter, speculation, and above all, gossip!

- Return phone calls and e-mails in a timely manner.

- Do your best to complete all work tasks as quickly and with as much quality as you can. Don't perceive any tasks to be too "trivial" for your best effort and creativity. Meet deadlines. If you, or your team, cannot meet a deadline, give as much notice to your superiors or customers as possible.

If you are the leader of a team, committee, or company, recognize that communication is one of your foremost responsibilities. Lead the way in establishing written policies and addressing boundary-setting issues. If you don't have an "answer" for a particular problem or need that may arise, don't make up one. Let your followers know that you are making the problem or need your top priority and that you will communicate answers as quickly as you have them—and then give them something specific and concrete to do in the meantime.

No company or committee likes employee turnover—it is costly, disruptive, and in many cases, primarily the fault of an employer who does not value his employees or treat all employees with a degree of consistency and fairness. Every person wants to have his or her dignity maintained, and to be treated with respect. Acknowledge the successes and achievements of the individuals in your organization (without playing favorites). Be sensitive to racial, age, and sexual differences within your employee or membership ranks. Avoid telling off-color or inappropriate jokes or stories. Praise the behavior you want to see continue.

At the same time, if problems arise, deal with them as quickly, decisively, and consistently as you can.

Develop a mindset that your job is not *truly* more important than the lowest job on the company hierarchy chart. Every person in an organization has a job to do and a role to fulfill, and failure at any level by any person becomes the "weak link" that can cause great harm. As the leader of a company, or division of a company, you may have a bigger salary and more people to supervise—and likely more authority within the company than most others—but your authority also has bigger *responsibilities*, and one of those foremost responsibilities is to role model the attitudes you want others in your group to have regarding quality, personal integrity, politeness and respect, and loyalty. Set realistic expectations for others, and they in turn will likely give you their best effort and loyalty.

Deal with sick time, worker's compensation, and general vacation schedules in an equitable manner. Recognize that having a WELLNESS program within your company or organization can be a great asset when it comes to energizing your people. Companies with a WELLNESS program nearly always report a lowering of sick-time hours, fewer injuries on the job, and greater morale and job satisfaction on the part of both employees and their supervisors. WELLNESS programs establish a general atmosphere of "being at one's best," and this can readily lead to a company or organization becoming its best as well!

If you lead your company to wellness, it will follow.

The Spill-over Effect of Pre-habilitation. When a person adopts a general perspective of pre-habilitation—in personal matters, in a family, and in work relationships—there is nearly always a spill-over effect. ALL of life seems to function in a more proactive, preventative manner. Problems are averted or avoided routinely in all sectors of life.

Notes about the INTELLECTUAL Dimension of Phase 3

1. Explore your spectrum of talents.

Every person is born with a set of talents and aptitudes. Most people have at least two major aptitudes, and a unique propensity for using them in various ways. Add to the mix a set of interests and dreams and the combinations are almost endless when it comes to what a person might become or accomplish in life.

Take time to explore your talents. You may want to revisit things that you "used to enjoy" as a child, or that you were told from birth that you were "good at." Recapture some of those old abilities and interests that may have gone dormant. In doing so, you likely will find new interests and new levels of fulfillment and joy.

2. Be on the alert for good learning opportunities.

Keep your antenna up at all times for interesting opportunities to add a skill to your resume or to gain information that seems interesting or vital to you for some reason. Seminars, conferences, retreats, short courses, and day-long information sessions abound! Take advantage of them.

3. Expand your circle of wise counselors and mentors.

Every person gets the best information and wisdom from a true *expert*—somebody who not only has information but EXPERIENCE.

In my opinion, everybody needs at least three experts feeding wise counsel into their life on a continual basis:

- A nutrition and fitness counselor or coach. Go to someone who truly has an understanding of what it takes to prevent illness and to maintain wellness.

- A good teacher or mentor, especially a person with experience and knowledge in an area associated with your foremost intellectual interests or career. This person should understand the nature of your work and be familiar with the financial constraints associated with it.

- A good "doctor" for your heart and soul—this might be a spiritual counselor or spiritual director, a pastor, or a person you know who has a depth of spiritual wisdom and experience in living out their beliefs.

Think BODY, SOUL (emotions and mind), and SPIRIT. Have an identifiable expert in each of these areas of your life!

Surround yourself with people who ARE
who you want to become.

Notes about the SPIRITUAL Dimension of Phase 3

Give back.

You will find tremendous fulfillment in life as you begin to "give back" to your community, church, and individuals who have a need you can meet.

Give more than money. Give your time and your talent. Become a role model or a mentor to the next generation. Offer your compassion and services to the elderly. Find a slot in a hospital or other area where you can be of real *service*.

Yes, you will be blessing others.

And yes, indeed, you will be *blessed* in return.

9

WELLNESS: A LIFESTYLE FOR THE REST OF YOUR LIFE

DEVELOPING A WELLNESS PLAN is not an exercise … it is not a course … it is an ongoing concept and plan for a way to LIVE the greatest, most fulfilling life possible.

The quest for wellness does not have an end point prior to death. It is something worthy of continual and diligent pursuit—because it *is* the fountain of the energy and strength to be and do all that you were created to be and do. It is the foremost key, in my opinion, to your living an "abundant life" on this earth and to amassing a full spectrum of eternal rewards.

We regularly use the number "10" in our culture as a number associated with perfection. The truth is, very few people will ever be a "10" in any category related to wellness, and if they do attain that rating, the perfection isn't likely to last very long. *Nobody* is a "10" in all areas of wellness. That does not mean, however, that we cannot aspire to that goal. The closer we get to a "10" the better! There's joy in the journey.

Why Make Wellness a Priority?

You will have to come up with your own answers to this question. Let me give you the seven reasons that I make a wellness program a priority:

1. I want to enjoy an enhanced quality of life every day of my life.

2. I want to get the most out of every day I live—do the most, experience the most, love others the best I can, and have the greatest influence I can have on what is right, good, just, and worthy of commitment in this life.

3. I want to be free of illness and disease, as much as possible.

4. I want to have a healthy mind, emotions, and spirit.

5. I want to be a role model worth emulating—to the next generation, as well as to my peers.

6. I want to fulfill the purpose for which I believe God has put me on this earth.

7. I want to build a life of *real* value by developing close friendships and loving family relationships, and by investing my time and resources in things that have

eternal value. In many ways, my pursuit of wellness *is* my outward expression that I inwardly value my life as a beloved child of God. It is my way of displaying honor to my Creator.

What do *you* say?

I encourage you to write down your reasons and keep this list in a place where you can refer to it often.

Continue to Kindle Your Spiritual Core

A spiritual life is intended to be just that ... *life*. It is expected to be a source of energy to all other aspects of your being. It is rooted in what you believe, and in your concept of eternity.

My faith is very important to me and I don't back down on its importance. At the same time, I never try to cram what I believe down another person's throat. Doing so can make another person bitter or resentful, which is the exact opposite outcome I desire!

Here are three principles that I have chosen to live by when it comes to my faith:

First, I let my faith-based values be my guide—both in what I say and in what I do. Positive words are empty if they don't result in positive deeds. One Bible writer referred to meaningless words as "clanging gongs." They hold noise but no benefit.

Second, I seek to speak always with a tone of love.

If you disagree with someone or if you are hurt by something a person says or does, it is certainly acceptable to say so ... but voice your words with a tone of kindness and respect. A judgmental, condemning, or angry tone will get you nowhere. Your loving tone of voice is likely to be remembered even more than any words you say.

Third, I *will* not compromise my morals.

Your display of moral character will be the foundation of your reputation in the eyes of others. Your morals are what *make* you a positive role model. They are what will influence your children more than anything else. They are what will win you "honor" and compel others to listen to your words that truly can help them experience earthly blessings and gain eternal rewards.

These three markers of my spiritual life are just as important to me today as they were yesterday, and I expect them to be important tomorrow and every day after that. In other words, there is never a day that I can foresee when I will NOT want to kindle my spiritual life.

That's the perspective I also have about wellness and wholeness.

Turn Hope into Expectancy

I have the opportunity to look into the eyes of thousands of people a year … sometimes in a corporate conference auditorium, sometimes in a church sanctuary, sometimes in an outdoor venue. The eyes are not always American eyes—at times they are African or Latino or Asian eyes.

What I nearly always see is a "look" in the eyes of my audience members that conveys, "I long for hope."

Hope for a better life.

Hope for greater wellness—which can also be hope for better health, hope for reconciled relationships, hope for more opportunity, and hope for a closer relationship with God.

Hope for positive change that might be both real and lasting.

My goal, of course, is to see that look of LONGING for hope change by the end of my seminar or presentation into a look of EXPECTANCY.

People not only want someone to say, "I think you can change." They want real tools and a how-to approach that includes specific goals and behaviors. These practical ways to ACT on hope turn their hopes into genuine EXPECTANCY.

What is your experience with this?

The Bible says that faith is believing and that our believing must be tied into believing *for something*. The fact that we can and do *believe* should be taken by us as evidence that the thing for which we are believing is possible. And if we have good reason to think that the thing for which we believe is GOOD for us, then we are in a position to believe for a miraculous change!

Choose to have hope.

Choose to believe that you can achieve a greater state of wellness.

Choose to believe that this is a good goal and one God desires for you.

And then act on your hope and get busy pursuing each of your wellness goals.

10

LET ME PROVE IT TO YOU

MY ADMONITION in this book is this: "Let me prove it to you!" I can and will.

In this book, I have given you lots of information and back-up examples that give evidence to WHY my wellness-coaching advice has worked for others and has a very high likelihood of working for *you*.

There is no proof, however, apart from you DOING what I am recommending. In essence:

The Proof Is In the Doing

And … that proof is not in MY doing, or in the doing of hundreds of people for whom I could offer testimonials of THEIR doing and THEIR results. The real *proof* is going to lie in YOUR developing a total Wellness Plan and making a diligent, consistent effort at implementing it in your own life.

I challenge you today …

Pursue WELLNESS.

Set your goals. Make your plan for achieving them.

And then take action. DO what you know is right to do FOR YOUR life and future.

Teach wellness to your children.

Role-model wellness to others with whom you are in contact.

Implement a wellness perspective in places where you work, socialize, and worship.

Let's enjoy WELLNESS together!

Share Your Story!

When you have implemented this Wellness Plan in your life, or in your family, company, or church, tell me your story to add to the "proof" that this plan works!

You can tell me your story at: *mark@live4e.com*

I'd love to hear it!

Yours for maximum health and wellness,

Dr. Mark